ROUTLEDGE LIBRARY EDITIONS:
PSYCHIATRY

Volume 24

COGNITIVE BEHAVIOURAL INTERVIEWING FOR ADULT DISORDERS

COGNITIVE BEHAVIOURAL INTERVIEWING FOR ADULT DISORDERS

A Practical Handbook

PETER H. WILSON, SUSAN H. SPENCE
AND DAVID J. KAVANAGH

Routledge
Taylor & Francis Group
LONDON AND NEW YORK

First published in 1989 by Routledge

This edition first published in 2019
by Routledge
2 Park Square, Milton Park, Abingdon, Oxon OX14 4RN

and by Routledge
711 Third Avenue, New York, NY 10017

Routledge is an imprint of the Taylor & Francis Group, an informa business

British Library Cataloguing in Publication Data
A catalogue record for this book is available from the British Library

ISBN: 978-1-138-60492-6 (Set)
ISBN: 978-0-429-43807-3 (Set) (ebk)
ISBN: 978-1-138-32472-5 (Volume 24) (hbk)
ISBN: 978-0-429-45073-0 (Volume 24) (ebk)

Publisher's Note
The publisher has gone to great lengths to ensure the quality of this reprint but points out that some imperfections in the original copies may be apparent.

Disclaimer
The publisher has made every effort to trace copyright holders and would welcome correspondence from those they have been unable to trace.

COGNITIVE BEHAVIOURAL INTERVIEWING FOR ADULT DISORDERS

A PRACTICAL HANDBOOK

PETER H. WILSON, SUSAN H. SPENCE
AND DAVID J. KAVANAGH

ROUTLEDGE

First published in 1989
by Routledge
11 New Fetter Lane, London EC4P 4EE
29 West 35th Street, New York, NY 10001

Typeset by Pat and Anne Murphy,
Highcliffe-on-Sea, Dorset
Printed and bound in Great Britain by
Mackays of Chatham PLC, Chatham, Kent

British Library Cataloguing in Publication Data

Wilson, Peter H
Cognitive behavioural interviewing for adult disorders
1. Medicine. Psychiatry. Interviewing — Manuals
I. Spence, Susan H. II. Kavanagh, David J.
616.89'0751

ISBN 0-415-00111-0
ISBN 0-415-00112-9 Pbk

To our present and past students
at The University of Sydney

Contents

1
Introduction

Aim and content of this book

The aim of this book is to provide guidelines for the conduct of initial interviews with people who present with some of the very common problems for which psychological assistance is sought. The book is intended to form a bridge between the numerous texts on behavioural assessment and those that review and describe the cognitive and behavioural treatments for psychological problems. Many of the texts on behavioural assessment place considerable emphasis on the assessment of the severity of the problems. Thus, they provide valuable information concerning the self-report, physiological and objective measurement procedures that the clinician may find useful in the assessment of many problems. The books on behavioural and cognitive therapies typically describe the treatment procedures that can be employed with the numerous disorders with which the clinician needs to deal. However, an important step in the process of assessment is the conduct of the initial interview in which information needs to be gathered from clients in a systematic, thorough, useful and economic manner. Such information, if well-collected, is essential for the specification of those aspects of the presenting problems that are important in designing appropriate and successful treatment interventions. The aim of this book is to assist the clinician in conducting initial interviews with clients who present with some of the most common problems.

The problems include depression, anxiety and phobias, headaches, insomnia, sexual problems, excessive consumption of alcohol and other drugs, social competence problems and obesity.

These problems are those which the student in clinical training is likely to meet in a typical outpatient setting in which a cognitive-behavioural approach is adopted. They span a range of areas including serious psychopathology, behavioural medicine, and problems of everyday living. It is hoped that detailed discussion of these problems might serve as a model for the design of interviews with people who present with other similar problems which we do not cover in this book, such as pain, obsessive-compulsive disorder or habitual behaviour problems. We have chosen to omit discussion of marital problems because of the need to consider additional complexities involved in such cases. There is a widespread view that standard interviews of the type presented here for other problems may best be avoided in the assessment of marital problems. Certain other problems such as anorexia nervosa, or psychotic disorders like schizophrenia or bipolar affective disorder have been omitted because they are more likely to be seen in inpatient units. While we have had to limit the focus of the book, we hope that certain general principles concerning the structure and content of cognitive-behavioural interviewing will be gleaned from the detailed examination of the selected topics, which will serve the clinician well in dealing with other problem areas.

This book is based on the assumptions that rational explanations exist for the causes of problems experienced as psychological disorders, that a knowledge of the likely causal processes is important for an adequate understanding of such disorders and that such knowledge, when applied to an individual case, will result in more efficacious and efficient treatment. These beliefs are consistent with a general experimental-clinical approach to psychological disorders, which implies that such disorders occur as a result of various behavioural, cognitive, social and physiological processes. This approach suggests that important distinctions can be made between various disorders in terms of their likely causality, and that, even within categories of disorders, there is a need to distinguish between possibly different psychological and physical processes that may play a causal, maintaining or ancillary role.

In each chapter, we will provide a summary of the current knowledge about a specific disorder, usually beginning with some discussion about the primary features that are generally considered to characterise the disorder and its potential subtypes, before going on to discuss the likely content of an initial interview. We have employed the diagnostic scheme presented in the Diagnostic and Statistical Manual of DSM-III (American Psychiatric Association,

1980) and its revision, DSM-III-R (1987). However, it ought to be noted that any classification system is an attempt by researchers and clinicians to bring about some order out of apparent chaos. Any such classification scheme reflects our ways of viewing the phenomena at a given point in time, and is subject to potential errors of perception, organisation and theory. Clinicians and students sometimes regard DSM-III as a stone tablet handed down to us from some omniscient authority. Such a view is likely to be dangerous if it prevents us from gaining new insights into the massive range of features that we meet in clinical practice. In this book, we use DSM-III-R as a starting point for the classification of some of the disorders under discussion, although this approach is not intended to imply complete acceptance of DSM-III-R. Thus, we will draw attention to potential inadequacies in this classification scheme where we consider that such views may be helpful to the reader.

What is cognitive-behavioural interviewing?

In this book we use the term 'cognitive-behavioural interviewing' to refer to the procedure by which information is obtained from a client that will assist in the identification of the presenting problem(s), the description of important aspects of the problems and the selection of appropriate treatment interventions. The term 'cognitive behavioural' is used to denote the general theoretical position from which this approach was derived. This term is being used in its broad sense, which includes consideration of overt behaviour, cognitive components and physiological activity. Throughout the book there is an acceptance of the theoretical importance of antecedents and consequences of *behaviour* and *thought* in the development and maintenance of psychological problems. We are in agreement with many other contemporary researchers in this field that cognitive processes are also relevant to an understanding of these problems (e.g. Bandura, 1977a; Mahoney, 1974; Meichenbaum, 1977), although we do not accept that such cognitive processes are necessarily the primary causative factors in all psychological problems.

The behavioural approach places considerable emphasis on the capacity for behaviour to be elicited by environmental cues. Thus, smoking may be elicited by the presence of cues previously associated with this behaviour such as the presence of an ash-tray, an advertisement or consumption of a cup of coffee. Likewise, it is possible that certain physical reactions such as those that are seen in anxiety may be elicited by environmental stimuli. A portion of the behavioural interview ought to be directed at the identification of cues that may be responsible for eliciting the problem behaviour. Some behaviour may be determined largely by the consequences with which it is followed. Thus, the occurrence of aversive stimuli consequent to the emission of a behaviour will tend to reduce the frequency of that behaviour, and the occurrence of appetitive stimuli will tend to increase the frequency of the behaviour. For each problem, we have discussed those aspects of the potential consequences that the clinician may need to examine in detail. For example, in discussing depression, we have drawn attention to the possibility that some depressive behaviour may be reinforced by the attention of significant others in the person's environment.

Triple-response modalities

The behavioural approach to assessment places emphasis on the need to examine three response modalities: overt behaviour, cognitive components and physiological activity. Overt behaviour includes objectively observable aspects of the problem, e.g. the number of drinks consumed per day, the frequency of panic attacks, engagement in certain activities. The cognitive components are the thoughts that precede, accompany or follow the occurrence of events or behaviours. Physiological activity refers to those features of the problem that involve some physiological change, e.g. perspiration, heart rate or respiration, or muscle tension. Many psychological problems involve more than one of these modalities. For example, a person with a public-speaking phobia may manifest avoidance of speaking situations, thoughts about appearing foolish prior to being in a speaking situation and an increase in heart rate when exposed to the speaking situation. Thus, assessment is directed at the evaluation of the level of all three modalities. Such information may be helpful in designing specific assessment devices and in selecting treatment components that are likely to be relevant to the manifestation of the problem in a given individual. Much of the research on the triple-response system has revealed a lack of agreement between the three modalities (e.g. Lang, 1968; Rachman & Hodgson, 1974). As a result of this observation, it has been proposed that each system may be controlled by different organismic and environmental factors. An alternative view is that the lack of agreement between the modalities could be expected to occur for several other reasons. First, the agreement between variables within one modality is often low, placing a restriction on the potential size of agreement between modalities. This point is particularly evident in the assessment of physiological activity, such as heart rate, muscle tension or galvanic skin response. Any one of these measures may provide a poor reflection of the physiological aspect of the particular problem under investigation in a particular individual. Second, the variety of assessments available under the rubric of cognitive measurement is also problematic in understanding the relationships between the three modalities. Assessment of cognitions may include self-observation of physiological activity or behaviour, causal attributions, self-ratings of symptom severity, self-efficacy judgments, distorted or irrational thinking and so forth. Many of these types of assessments can be conducted in several different ways and at different points in time in relation to the behaviour. Thus, the failure to find agreement between physiological, cognitive and behavioural modalities may be as much a reflection of the lack of agreement within modalities as it is a reflection of the operation of different systems. In this book, we have chosen, with the above qualification, to preserve the traditional focus on the triple-response modalities as an approach to assessment. Since the primary subject of the book is interviewing, our comments on the triple-assessment are mostly limited to the client's *observations* of their physiological, cognitive and behavioural functioning.

An important aspect of the cognitive and behavioural approaches is the emphasis on the evaluation of the present difficulties and circumstances of the person. The present-focus will often help to clarify the nature of the problem, and will generally be useful in providing clear targets for the intervention. It is very helpful to explore carefully the most recent instance of the occurrence of the problem while the details can be retrieved easily. Other instances that are worthy of detailed discussion include any particularly distressing or traumatic occasions. However, it is also necessary to obtain an appropriate amount of information about the person's previous history, and, in particular, the development of the problem for which help is being sought. Such information may provide useful insights into possible causal factors that may be of assistance in the design of interventions.

One theme that permeates this book is an acceptance of the hypothetico-deductive approach to assessment. In our provision of background information about each problem, we have attempted to summarise the principal theoretical and descriptive details that are necessary to achieve an understanding of the likely complexities of each problem. This approach is intended to result in the reader being able to identify those features of the presenting problem that may be useful in tailoring an individual treatment programme. For example, in the chapter on insomnia, attention is drawn to both the stimulus-control and the hyperarousal theories, and to the kind of information that would be pertinent to the identification of either processes as may occur in a given person. Thus, the clinician might obtain information that suggests the involvement of poor stimulus control as a basis for insomnia in a particular client, and would design an appropriate treatment programme accordingly. Admittedly, not all problems are amenable to such distinctive conceptualisations, and there is considerably more research needed concerning the prediction of treatment outcome and the matching of clients to treatments.

It is important to outline here some of the more general issues that may arise in the initial interview prior to discussion of individual problems. Thus, we will now turn to consideration of the overall structure and procedure of the initial interview, emphasising the clinical skills that are important to the application of the guidelines presented in the remainder of the text.

Some general caveats

In order to provide detailed discussion about each of the selected problems, it has been necessary to isolate each one within a separate chapter. However, the clinician needs to be aware that many clients will present with more than one problem, making it necessary to conduct investigations of each problem either separately or in some kind of joint fashion as the need arises. For example, a person who presents with depressive problems may also exhibit difficulties in social situations. A complete assessment would involve an investigation of both areas. In many places, we indicate the common concurrence of problems and we suggest that the reader refers to another chapter in this book for more details.

It should also be noted that a distinction can be drawn between those problems for which clients present themselves for treatment and other problems that the therapist may judge to be present in the course of the interview(s). We have generally commenced each guide to the conduct of the interview under the assumption that a client will have indicated the presence of certain problems either at the point of initial contact or very early in the interview. However, with minimal alterations, the clinician could conduct an interview with clients for whom he/she suspects the presence of a particular problem that has not been clearly stated by the client. For the most part, a modification of the opening questions might be needed to deal with the latter situation.

The interviewing guidelines have been constructed so that important aspects of each problem are covered. However, we would like to stress that each guide ought to be employed in a flexible manner, consistent with good clinical practice. The order of questions will need to be altered to suit most clinical situations. Some questions will need to be followed up by other detailed examination of issues not covered in this book. It may be necessary to abandon this style of interviewing altogether in some cases, e.g. with a highly distressed or suicidal person. It would also be necessary to extend interviewing over several sessions in many cases. *We cannot over-emphasise the need to incorporate this material into a general interviewing format, and to avoid rigidly adhering to the guidelines.* In many situations, the clinician might find it useful to go back over the interview guide after conducting an initial interview, in order to check whether all the potentially important information has been obtained.

Interviewing skills

The aim of an initial interview is to obtain information from the client about his or her problems in a comprehensive, efficient, systematic and humane manner. Not surprisingly, there are numerous skills involved in conducting interviews that meet these ideals. Throughout this book, we have placed considerable emphasis on the first three of these goals, and at this point we would like to focus on those aspects of the interview that call upon the interpersonal skills of the clinician to a very considerable extent. Our belief is that while the technical skills are necessary, they are unlikely to be sufficient if the clinician is unable to interact with the client in an encouraging, supportive and professional manner. The clinician needs to possess good listening skills in order to understand what the client is saying and experiencing, and good communication skills in order to convey this understanding to the client in an appropriate and constructive way. These skills, including the ability to express empathy, acceptance and support, can be manifested in the selection and wording of questions, the timing of questions in the interview, the feedback of your understanding of the client's feelings and even in moments of silence. One reason for avoiding the rigid use of our interviewing guides is that such use would imply a lack of ability to respond flexibly and skilfully to the enormous variety of circumstances that are likely to arise in interviews with clients, even with those who ostensibly share the same general problem. At this stage, we will provide a brief overview of the main interpersonal skills involved in conducting clinical interviews and illustrate how these skills might be put to good effect.

Listening skills

It is important to convey that you are interested in listening to the person and are attending to the subtle nuances of their expression. Part of this skill involves non-verbal aspects such as erect but relaxed body posture, an appropriate degree of eye contact and a responsive facial expression. Care should be taken to ensure that the seating arrangement and distance is likely to be comfortable for the person. When the client is talking, it is important to wait until you think that the person has completely finished before you respond. Often, a slight pause will allow the client to offer additional information or to express more sensitive matters. It is important to ensure that you understand the client's experiences and feelings as the interview unfolds. If you pay close attention to what the client is saying, a question almost certainly will arise that may help to clarify any area of confusion. If you remain uncertain, it is best to seek clarification by saying something like: 'I'm not sure that I have this right, but as I understand it . . . is that correct?' This kind of statement conveys a sense of concern about the accuracy of your own understanding, and would generally be reassuring to the person. The clinician also needs to be aware of the significance or meaning of the client's comments, and to make a mental note of potential areas to follow up later if you would rather not interrupt the flow of material at the time. If it becomes necessary to change the topic for some period, a few words of explanation of the relevance of this area can be very helpful, while at the same time you should assure the client that you will return to the matter under discussion at a later point in time. Listening skills also include the use of careful observation of changes in the client's level of comfort when discussing different issues. One needs to notice changes in voice quality, facial expression, eye contact and movements of hands or legs. Such changes in non-verbal aspects of the communication may suggest areas of greater emotional significance, which could be followed up in more detail.

Empathy, acceptance and support

The term *empathy* refers to the conveyance to the client of your understanding of the feelings expressed and the experiences described from the client's point of view. It is not simply a matter of saying 'yes, I understand', but may involve paraphrasing the essential meaning of the previous statement, or summarising the main content of a broader set of material and drawing out any main connecting themes. It is also important to convey *acceptance* of the client's reactions and feelings without personal, moral or cultural judgment. Acceptance can be conveyed by avoiding evaluative expressions, either implicitly or explicitly. Care also needs to be taken in the wording of certain questions that avoid the implication that you hold certain general social prejudices. For example, in asking people about their sexual relationships or experiences, one should leave open the possibility that the person has had homosexual relationships rather than assuming that such relationships will always be heterosexual. If you convey that you are evaluating the client, it is rather unlikely that the client will reveal very sensitive or distressing matters. *Support* is a difficult concept to define, but can be considered to include the general demeanour of the therapist in encouraging the clients to express their feelings and concerns. The style of the interviewer should be one of patience, warmth and attentiveness. It is important to convey that you can be relied upon for clear and helpful advice and encouragement by remaining unruffled and professional even when things get difficult.

Types of questions

It is possible to classify questions broadly into closed or open-ended categories. Closed questions are those to which the only likely response is 'yes' or 'no', such as, 'did you feel anxious when . . . ?' Open questions are those to which the person can respond more freely, such as 'how did you feel when . . . ?' Both types of questions have their place, and the ideal interview technique involves a blend of open questions (to obtain the maximum amount of information with a minimum of bias due to the content of the question itself) and closed questions (to provide specific answers to precise questions of fact). In the interview guides, you will find a mixture of questions of both types, reflecting the need for a blend of specific and general questioning about different topics. There may be occasions when you realise that a more open question was required after asking a closed question. In such situations, it is often helpful to ask the question again with some slight modification. It is especially important to ascertain whether the person has actually answered the question that you intended, or whether the client has answered 'another question' due either to a misunderstanding of the question as stated or to some other factor such as avoidance of certain issues.

Your use of language is an important tool in the interviewing procedure. In this regard, it is important to select words and expressions carefully, so that you convey your meaning clearly to the client. A part of this skill involves the avoidance of jargonistic phrases or words, such as 'stimuli', 'reinforcement', 'cognitions', 'self-statements' and so forth. It is also necessary to judge the level of vocabulary that is appropriate for an individual client, and to tailor your language accordingly.

We have only been able to provide a very brief overview of some of the main interpersonal aspects of interviewing. It is recommended that the reader consult such texts as Nay (1979), Tyler (1969), Kanfer and Saslow (1969) and Truax and Carkuff (1967) for more detailed discussion of many of the clinical skills, issues and procedures involved in clinical interviewing.

Planning the interview

We have taken the view that it is helpful to plan or structure most interviews in order to obtain a comprehensive and elucidating view of the problem in an efficient manner. The importance of the structure is that it helps the clinician to remember to cover potentially important areas in a systematic manner that is likely to lead to the identification of significant factors involved in the cause and maintenance of the problem, and hence to the design of an individually tailored treatment programme. Several general principles are worthy of note here, especially if one is to be able to transfer the application of this procedure to problems not covered in this book.

One feature of the plan of each chapter is the adoption of the SORC approach, advocated by Goldfried and Sprafkin (1976). SORC is an acronym for stimulus–organism–response–consequences, reflecting the importance of investigating the role of antecedent stimuli (S), physiological state and past learning (O) and consequences that follow a given behaviour (C) in understanding the factors that may influence the occurrence of the problematic behaviour or 'response' (R), the theoretical significance of which has been discussed previously. Thus, the reader will note that a structure underlies each interview in which there is movement through each of these areas. The order of discussion may vary somewhat, depending on the circumstances and the type of problem being considered. Of course, a great deal of time is spent on the discussion of the definition of the principal presenting problem. Thus, attention is given to assessment of severity of the problem. Severity can often be considered in terms of frequency, intensity and duration, although additional factors, such as the extent to which the person is limited in work, social or recreational activities, are also relevant to this judgment.

A second feature of the structure is the emphasis on the history of the problem. It is important to identify any events that may be associated with the early development of the problem, and any changes in its course over time. Questions concerning periods in which the problem has either improved or worsened can be helpful in identifying causal factors. It is important to obtain details of the events and circumstances surrounding any periods of change in either direction. For example, if it discovered that a person's sleep difficulties improved during a holiday, one might further explore the reasons for this change that could be due to alteration in stimulus control or to removal from stresses (or other factors). Detailed investigation of this period and other similar occasions may help to determine the most likely causal processes. As noted above, it is important not to ignore the person's general history. One would be particularly looking out for important key life events, especially as they relate to the present problems.

General background information

There are certain areas that a clinician would cover in almost any initial interview. These include general personal information such as age, occupation, education, marital status, family details, recreational interests, developmental history, duration and course of the presenting problem(s), types of previous treatments and response and any other relevant information. Such information might be obtained either at the beginning of the interview, or at some appropriate point in the course of the session.

General information is important for several reasons. First, the information may reveal important personal and historical factors that may be helpful in understanding the aetiology of the problem. The hypotheses developed by the clinician may be discussed with the client, who may be reassured that the problem has some rational explanation. Second, an understanding of the development of the problem may be useful in the formulation of a treatment programme. Third, there may be aspects of the person's background and history that may help to reveal assets and resources, or limitations and deficits that may affect the decisions made about the nature of the treatment programme.

Beginning the interview

The precise way in which you begin an interview will vary, depending upon the circumstances and the apparent state of the client at that time. Often, you will wish to introduce yourself and to explain that the purpose of the interview is to discover the ways in which you can help the person with the problems for which they have come to the clinic/hospital/treatment centre. A fairly general, open-ended question as in the following example will ordinarily be an appropriate type of question with which to commence:

In what way can I help you?

or

What is the reason that you made an appointment to see me?

After receiving a response to this initial question, you might go on to ask another very general question, such as:

Can you tell me more about that?

The history of the problem and major life events represents a major area of exploration in the initial interview(s). In particular, the clinician should look for any conjunction of events and problematic behaviour that may be suggestive of aetiological connections. A strategy that is often helpful in dealing with the mass of historical information that is often obtained at this point is to draw up a time-line of key events indicating the year of their occurrence.

When did you first notice that . . . was a problem for you?
Can you tell me about how it began or about the first time that you noticed it?
How has it changed over time?
Has there ever been a period when it improved quite a lot, or went away?
Can you tell me more about that time?

Find out more details of about that period, including significant events, etc.

What is the worst that it has been for you?

Find out more details of about that period, including significant events, etc.

When did you first start to think that you might get some help for . . . ?
Why was that?

At this stage, you might wish to commence the more detailed questions concerning the nature of the problem, as indicated in the subsequent chapters. The remaining questions suggested below are not necessarily placed in any important order. Such questions may need to be interspersed with the other questions contained in the detailed analysis of the problem.

Recent life events

A review of recent life events may be helpful as a means of identifying possible aetiological factors. The following questions provide a guide to this area:

Let's take a moment to review the events of the past year or so.
Have there been any important events that have taken place in your life over the last year?

Any events that are mentioned could be followed by a series of questions such as the following:

Can you tell me what happened in more detail?
What was the cause of . . . ? (*referring to the event*)
How did you react to /cope with /deal with . . . ? (*referring to the event*)

In case some events have been forgotten, it is useful to go through a short list:

Have there been any difficulties at work?
What about family difficulties?

Have there been any illnesses or deaths amongst friends or family?
Have there been any other difficulties?

History and present circumstances

The exploration of the person's general history and present life circumstances is seen as crucial to the conduct of initial interviews. In the following section, we have provided an outline of the kinds of questions that might be asked to cover such broad areas. Some of the information may have been obtained during the earlier parts of the interview and, of course, these sections would be omitted at this point. Other questions may not be appropriate under all circumstances. However, the following set of questions should be a helpful guide to the areas of most relevance.

We have spent quite a bit of time discussing the reasons for your visit here, and I am now starting to get a general picture of the situation, but it might be helpful at this stage if we discuss some more general areas — it will help me get to know more about you and may help me to understand more about the problems for which you have sought help. Let's start with some fairly general points, for example:
What kind of work do you do?
How long have you been doing that job?
Have you had any jobs prior to this one?
Can you tell me about these jobs?
Do you enjoy your work?
What are the things you like most about work?
What do you like least?
What age are you? *or* When were you born?
Where were you born?
Where did you spend your early years?
Have you lived anywhere else?
When did you arrive in . . . (*present location*)?
How do you find it here?
Where did you go to school?
What level of school did you reach?
How did you find school?
Are you married/presently involved in a relationship?
How long have you been married/involved in this relationship?

Obviously other questions may be appropriate in some circumstances, such as questions about divorce, separation, previous relationships or marriages.

If relevant:

What kind of work does your wife/husband/partner do?

Do you have any children?

Can you tell me about them — their ages and so forth?

Further explore whether these children live at home, and whether any other people such as relatives or friends live in the same home.

How much time do you spend with your family?

Is this satisfactory to you?

How would you describe your relationship with your wife/husband/partner?

What about your children — how do you get along with them?

Similarly, for any important others such as parents or in-laws:

What kinds of things do you like to do in your spare time?

Do you have any special hobbies or interests?

Selecting some of these activities:

How much time do you spend . . . ? *or* How often do you do . . . ?

How much time do you spend with friends or other relatives?

Are you happy with this amount of time?

Do you have any particularly close friends?

Find out details, such as the number of such friends, amount of contact, degree of satisfaction, etc.

Do you belong to any religion?

You might find out some details about the practice of any religious beliefs, the influence of religion on the person's life, etc.

Treatment history

An investigation of previous treatments is often particularly useful. For example, knowledge of a previously good response to treatment with a subsequent relapse could help direct the clinician towards using certain relapse-prevention strategies or to a reconceptualisation of the critical factors involved in the development of the problem. Similarly, the failure of previous interventions will alert the clinician to carefully consider the use of comparable procedures. In such cases, it would be especially useful to discuss the details of the content of the previous treatment, and the person's judgment about the reasons for failure. The following questions might be useful.

Have you received any treatment before for this problem?

Find out details, such as when, where, from whom, etc.

What effect did that treatment have at the time?

Look for immediate effects, then explore the changes that took place after treatment.

Why do you think that this/these treatment(s) failed to help you?

Have you received treatment for any other problems?

Once again find out the full details.

Have you had any health problems in the last few years?

If yes:

What kinds of problems have you had?

Have you ever been admitted to hospital for treatment?

Obtain details of the nature of the treatment, cause of the hospitalisation, effects, etc.

Are you taking any medication at present?

If yes:

Can you tell me the names of these medications?

Go through each one finding out the details of the dosage, reasons for taking them and their effects.

General

Several other areas of inquiry are often fruitful. Ordinarily, one would want to know why the client has sought treatment at this particular point in time, since there may have been some significant triggering factor such as pressure from spouse, impending or recent events, or some other precipitant. It is also helpful to know if the person has told his/her spouse or close friends that he/she is coming to see you since this information might cast light on the quality of significant relationships. The expectations that the person has about the content and outcome of treatment is a further area of inquiry that ought to be explored. In the following guide, we have attempted to provide demonstration questions designed to cover these areas. The section also begins with clarification of the main goal of any therapeutic intervention. This set of questions would be most appropriately placed at the end of the interview, since the areas of inquiry would lead easily into a discussion about the type of treatment that you could offer, clarification of the likely outcome and possibly, the establishment of a specific contract.

What do you see as the main difficulty with which you want help at the present time?

Are there any other things that you would add to that?

Why do you think that you have to come along here for help with . . . at this particular point in time?

How did you come to find about our clinic/services?

Have you told your spouse/partner about coming here?

If yes:
  How did he/she react?
If no:
  Why not?
  Have you told anyone else?

Concluding the interview

  How do you feel about coming here today?
  Has it turned out to be what you expected?
If yes:
  In what ways?
If no:
  How is it different?
  How confident are you that you can get over this difficulty by coming here?

At this point you might explore reasons for confidence or lack of it. One aim of this discussion is to reach an understanding of the client's motivation for treatment. You may need to further discuss this issue, clarifying the likely expectation of success and the duration of time that may be needed to reach that goal. Care should be taken to see that the client leaves with a positive (but realistic) expectation about the outcome. If either you or the client consider that the treatments that you can offer are inappropriate for the particular problems, this point should be carefully discussed with the person, and a referral should be made to a suitable person or agency. In concluding the interview, it is also important to convey to the client your understanding of the main aspects of their problems, and to summarise the principal points as you see them. Some indication of the kind of approach that you would take to help the person may also be reassuring. The client's reactions to the nature of treatment should be explored in detail. An important point to convey is the collaborative nature of the approach in which the client can assist in deciding how to determine priorities in treatment and how to achieve the stated goals.

Specific assessment methods

In each chapter we have presented some details of the kinds of assessment devices that can be employed to assess the severity of the various problems under consideration. One purpose of the initial interview is to provide a sufficient definition of the presenting problems so that further detailed assessment can be undertaken. Thus, the reader will frequently need to conduct a further evaluation of the severity of the problems using standard assessment methods. Such assessment devices will also be useful in the continuous monitoring of progress and in the evaluation of the outcome of treatment. To meet these needs, we have made mention of the major assessment procedures, and indicated the uses to which they might be put. We have placed emphasis on the most widely accepted self-report and objective measures. However, the reader is urged to consult texts on behavioural assessment and original articles for further detailed discussion of the psychometric properties of these instruments. Such general texts include those by Hersen and Bellack (1981), Cimminero, Calhoun and Adams (1977), or Barlow (1981).

Often the clinician will find that it is helpful to develop a daily monitoring form in order to enable the client to keep records of certain aspects of the problem in the period between the first and second sessions. This form of assessment can assist in the measurement of the frequency and intensity of the problem, and may yield valuable information about the factors that influence its occurrence. This procedure also reinforces the collaborative nature of the therapeutic endeavour. For example, a person who presents with headaches might be asked to keep records on a standard form on which a rating is made of the severity and duration of the pain, its location and any events that preceded the headache. Such monitoring is particularly useful for discrete problems such as instances of heightened anxiety, habitual behaviours, social difficulties, insomnia, consumption of alcohol and cigarette smoking. Similar procedures can be adapted for less discrete problems such as mood disorders or general anxiety by asking the person to record the intensity of such feelings on a 10-point scale at certain times of the day. It is often useful to have the clients record other aspects of their experiences, such as their activity throughout the day. We would suggest that the clinician goes over such forms with the client very carefully, using that day or the previous day as an example, in order to clarify the nature of the task to the client and to determine whether the client will have any difficulty in completing the form. Although we have provided examples of these types of forms, such monitoring devices can be individually tailored to cope with the specific needs of the client. Some clients prefer to have less structure, and for these clients, a diary format may be a satisfactory alternative.

Treatment

The main aim of this book is to provide assistance to the clinician in the conduct of initial interviews, rather than to describe the treatment of psychological problems. However, at various points we have suggested that certain information about the person may lead to the likely use of a specific treatment approach. Thus, at the end of each chapter we have provided a very brief overview of the major treatment options for each problem area. This section is intended primarily to direct the reader to other material in which the treatment procedures will be described in detail. We have also included references to recent papers that provide reviews of the efficacy of treatments for each problem. For more general information on cognitive and behaviour therapy, the reader should also consult several of the major texts in this area such as Craighead, Kazdin & Mahoney (1981) and Kendall & Hollon (1979).

Structure of interview in review

Based on the information presented above, it is now possible to provide an overview of the main elements that need to be present in most interviews. These elements include:

General information — age, marital status, occupation, educational history, religion, family details, interest and hobbies, social activity.

Developmental information — key life events.

Health — medical history, current medication (diet and exercise may also be relevant on occasions).

History of the problem — duration, changes in severity, nature of onset, development.

Nature of the problem — chief presenting problem defined specifically, other problems.

Features of the problem — severity (frequency, intensity, duration), physiological, cognitive and behavioural features.

Aetiology — antecedents, consequences, physiological, current precipitants.

Maintenance — positive reinforcers for occurrence, avoidance, social context.

Previous treatment — types, reactions, initial and long-term responses.

Other — motivation, expectation of outcome.

In the following chapters, we will assume that the information of a general kind that has been discussed in this introduction will be covered elsewhere in your interview. Thus, we will place most of our emphasis on the gathering of specific information that may be particularly pertinent to the problem that forms the topic of each chapter.

2
Fear and Anxiety Problems

Introduction

When people say that they feel afraid or anxious, they base this partly on an assessment of their physiological state. In general, this involves a reaction by the sympathetic nervous system, in which the body is prepared for vigorous muscular activity and possible physical injury. It usually includes: (a) accelerated heart rate and an increase in the volume of blood being pumped with each beat; (b) redistribution of blood flow from the skin and gut to the muscles and brain; (c) sweating, which triggers a rise in skin conductivity; (d) more rapid respiration; (e) a rise in the level of haemoglobin, coagulants, lymphocyte cells and sugar in the blood; (f) inhibition of salivation, stomach contractions, digestive secretion and intestinal peristalsis; (g) inhibition of sexual excitement; and (h) dilation of pupils and inhibition of tear glands. In extreme reactions, bladder and anal sphincter control may be lost. The reaction is often accompanied by a rise in muscle tension throughout the body, so that a person experiencing chronic anxiety will frequently complain of fatigue and muscular discomfort.

There are substantial individual differences in the patterning of somatic arousal, so that no single measure can fully represent the extent of somatic response across individuals (Lacey & Lacey, 1968). Different people may also focus on different aspects of their reactions in estimating their fear response. To complicate matters further, physiological responses are not the only data on which people base judgments of their anxiety or fear level. They also take into account their subjective interpretations of these responses, their beliefs about the situation they are facing and their inferred ability to deal with its challenges. When people view a situation as potentially dangerous and doubt their ability to control the threat, they interpret their physiological reaction as fear (Bandura, 1986). To resolve the problem, they often leave the situation as soon as possible, and may avoid it in future. Severe reactions of this kind are labelled phobias. However, people differ in the patterning of physiological, cognitive–emotional and behavioural aspects to phobic reactions, so that some show mainly avoidance and others may still confront the situation but have an exaggerated physiological response. As a result, measurement of any one aspect may not capture the degree or the pattern of the problem for a particular individual (Lang, 1971). This has led Lang (1977) to put forward a tripartite theory of fear that incorporates the somatic, subjective and behavioural aspects. While this confuses the cognitive-behavioural experience of fear with behavioural coping strategies that the person mobilises (Bandura, 1986), Lang's recommendation to assess all three of his problem aspects is well made.

Until recently, the predominant approach to phobias within experimental psychology has been the two-factor theory of Mowrer (1947). In this view, the phobic stimulus obtains noxious properties by classical conditioning, and avoidance behaviour is reinforced by reductions in anxiety due to withdrawal of the feared stimulus. However, this theory does not account well for more recent experimental data (Rachman, 1976, 1977). Classical conditioning via direct experience with the phobic stimulus is not necessary for the acquisition of fear and avoidance: Fears can be acquired through observation of others or by description of their experience (Bandura, 1977b; Bandura & Rosenthal, 1966). Nor is autonomic arousal necessary for the acquisition and maintenance of avoidance learning (Wynne & Solomon, 1955). Treatment of avoidance does not require a prior reduction in anxiety (Bandura, Blanchard & Ritter, 1969), and treatment-induced changes in avoidance are often poorly correlated with reductions in arousal (Leitenberg, Agras, Butz & Wincze, 1971). Indeed, it is difficult to see how a reduction in arousal can act as a reinforcer for avoidance, since the behaviour often occurs before the autonomic response occurred (Bandura, 1986).

Bandura (1977b, 1986) proposes an alternative view that displaces anxiety from its role as the primary cause of avoidant behaviour, and instead, sees the anxiety and behaviour as co-effects. The predominant mediator of each is the person's self-efficacy, or perceived capability in dealing with prospective situations. When we feel unable to deal with a demanding situation, we are less likely to engage in it, and if we do make an attempt, we invest less effort and give up more easily (Bandura, 1977b, 1982). We also see ourselves as being vulnerable to the consequences of the failure to meet situational demands, and it is the prospect of these consequences of inefficacy, rather than the situation itself, that is seen as the primary basis of our emotional arousal (Bandura, Reese & Adams, 1982; Williams & Watson, 1985). If self-efficacy is the central mechanism for phobic reactions, this accounts for the fact that emotional arousal is not required for the acquisition or maintenance of the phobia. Instead, the focus shifts to the ways in which self-efficacy is undermined or increased. Consistent with the effectiveness of performance-based treatments for phobias (Emmelkamp, 1979), performance accomplishments are the strongest information source of self-efficacy (Bandura, 1977b). Apart from the salience of the direct experience, these accomplishments confirm to us that we have the requisite skills for the situation. But performance accomplishments are not the only source for self-efficacy judgements. People also use vicarious experiences, verbal communications and assessments of their emotional arousal to develop self-efficacy judgements. This helps to explain the vicarious acquisition of phobia, and advances a theoretical explanation for treatments such as symbolic modelling and systematic desensitisation (Bandura, 1977b). In view of the predictive utility and determinative role of self-efficacy, its measurement is an important feature of the assessment.

Both the two-factor theory of Mowrer and the social-cognitive account of Bandura are potentially modified by the notion of biological preparedness advanced by Seligman & Hager (1972). Preparedness theory attempts to account for the differential incidence of particular fears by advancing the idea of genetic susceptibility or preparedness for certain associations that have evolutionary significance for the species. At this point, evidence for the hypothesis remains inconclusive at best (Delprato, 1980). A number of apparently supportive studies confound stimulus qualities of the objects such as unpredictability and uncontrollability with their evolutionary significance (Bandura, 1986). So, for example, the behaviour of an inanimate electric cord is viewed as more predictable than the slitherings of a snake, even though the cord may be objectively more dangerous. Modelling of fear responses and cultural beliefs also frequently confound with hereditary factors (Bandura, 1986). For our purpose, the argument appears to have little significance. Although prepared stimuli may be more resistant to extinction (Ohman, Eriksson & Olofsson, 1975), preparedness has little value in predicting response to treatment (De Silva, Rachman & Seligman, 1977; Zafiropoulou & McPherson, 1986).

Types of fear and anxiety reactions

DSM-III-R (American Psychiatric Association, 1987) divides anxiety disorders into (1) Panic disorder; (2) Agoraphobia without history of panic disorder; (3) Social phobia; (4) Simple phobia; (5) Obsessive–compulsive disorder; (6) Post-traumatic stress disorder; (7) Generalised anxiety disorder; and (8) Anxiety disorder not otherwise specified, a residual anxiety disorder category. This chapter will not examine obsessive–compulsive disorder, and will focus particularly on panic and phobias.

Panic and agoraphobia

Panic attacks are episodes of intense physiological arousal that have a rapid onset and usually last less than 15 minutes, although some can extend over several hours. Features may include: (a) dyspnea (shortness of breath) or smothering sensations; (b) dizziness, unsteady feelings or faintness (i.e. feeling one is about to faint; (c) palpitations or accelerated heart rate; (d) trembling or shaking; (e) sweating; (f) choking; (g) nausea or abdominal distress; (h) depersonalisation or derealisation; (i) numbness or tingling sensations (parasthesias); (j) hot or cold flashes; (k) chest pain or discomfort; (l) fear of dying; and (m) fear of going crazy, or doing something uncontrolled during an attack (DSM-III-R, 1987, p. 238). For panic disorder, DSM-III-R requires one or more occasions when at least four of these features began suddenly and increased in intensity within ten minutes of the first symptom. Panic can occur in conjunction with a range of phobias and with other psychological problems (Dittrich, Houts & Lichstein, 1983). For DSM-III-R panic disorder, at some time in the disturbance one or more panic attacks that were not related to phobic situations must have occurred. The criteria also stipulate that four attacks must have occurred over a four-week period, or that one or more attacks were followed by at least a month of a persistent fear of having another attack.

Many of the features of panic attacks frequently appear to be related to the perceived difficulty in breathing, which the person tries to correct by hyperventilating (Franklin, 1984; Garssen, Van Veenendaal & Bloemink, 1983). Excessive oxygen may produce feelings of unreality, dizziness and faintness (Rapee, Mattick & Murrell, 1986), and the person's cognitive/emotional response triggers the remaining symptoms. Panic attacks typically do not result in loss of consciousness, despite the sensations of faintness: Actual fainting tends to be restricted to blood-illness-injury phobias (Connolly, Hallam & Marks, 1976) and is a reaction to a sudden drop in heart rate and blood pressure. Depersonalisation and derealisation also occur outside panic episodes, and are seen in around 13 per cent of a control population (Buglass, Clarke, Henderson, Kreitman & Presley, 1977). The incidence among agoraphobics is 30 to 50 per cent (Buglass *et al.*, 1977; Harper & Roth, 1962). Fear of dying is often related to the sensations of panic, being misperceived as evidence of a life-threatening illness. The physiological events are usually much less intense than they are perceived. For example, the increase in heart rate is substantially less than the rise after moderate exercise (Lader & Mathews, 1970). An oversensitivity to the sensations often results in episodes being triggered by non-phobic events such as hot weather, exercise or even hunger. The range of precipitants can contribute to the difficulty sufferers have in predicting high-risk situations.

Similar symptoms to a panic attack can be generated by a variety of physical conditions, including hypoglycemia (low blood sugar), caffeinism, amphetamine intoxication, withdrawal from barbiturates, hyperthyroidism, Menière's disease (vertigo), paroxysmal tachycardia, angina pectoris, anaphylaxsis (severe allergic reaction), pheochromocytoma (adrenal tumour), post-concussional syndrome and asthma. DSM-III-R excludes from panic disorder any symptoms that are sustained by known organic factors. One commonly associated condition that is not excluded by DMS-III-R is mitral valve prolapse (MVP), which is a structural dysfunction of the heart. MVP occurs in 40 to 50 per cent of people who have panic episodes, as against around 10 per cent of controls (Foa, Steketee & Young, 1984). Evidence is now accumulating that there is a genetic risk factor for panic disorder (Crowe, Noyes, Pauls & Slyman, 1983; Torgerson, 1983), perhaps through one or more of the predisposing conditions above. Unfortunately, diagnosis and treatment of a physiological contributor to a panic disorder does not necessarily relieve the anticipatory anxiety concerning the attacks (Klein, 1981). Psychological assessment and treatment may still be required.

In agoraphobia, the primary concern of the person is usually the occurrence of a panic attack, which is regarded as a catastrophic event (Goldstein & Chambless, 1978). This concern is often termed a 'fear of fear', and in self-efficacy terms, the crucual performance skill is control of the anxiety reaction. External situations became more problematic as they increase the perceived risk of the panic or make it more difficult to control, or intensify the negative consequences from failure. Because of the strong association between agoraphobia and panic, DSM-III-R now encompasses the majority of agoraphobic reactions in a subcategory of panic disorder (panic disorder with agoraphobia). Around 60 per cent of agoraphobics would fall into this category (Harper & Roth, 1962; Linton & Estock, 1977). Agoraphobia without a history of panic disorder is encoded separately.

Agoraphobia (literally a 'fear of the market place') often does involve fear and avoidance of streets and large open spaces (Marks, 1970). Other commonly feared situations include being in crowds, especially if escape is restricted. So, for example, the person frequently has problems in supermarket or cinema queues, in restaurants or when sitting away from the aisle in cinemas and churches. Being confined in a hairdresser's or dentist's chair, in public transport or in an elevator is also likely to be problematic. Generally, feared situations are worse when agoraphobics are alone, in unfamiliar surroundings, when far from safety or medical assistance or when restricted to the situation for a longer period. So, anxiety in a car may be exacerbated by traffic jams, bridges or tunnels, and by travelling longer distances. The fear is likely to peak at about the middle of the journey or at the furthest distance from a hospital.

Agoraphobics constitute 50 to 80 per cent of people who seek help for phobias (Foa *et al.*, 1984). While many fears are more commonly reported by women (Geer, 1965; Hersen, 1973), the gender difference is especially pronounced in agoraphobia, where 88 per cent were women in one large British survey (Burns & Thorpe, 1977). In some studies, the mean age of onset is in the mid-twenties (e.g. Sheehan, Sheehan & Minichiello, 1981), although other studies have found a bimodal distribution within a second peak in the late teens after leaving school (Marks & Gelder, 1966; Mendel & Klein, 1969). The typical agoraphobic is a married unemployed woman (Vandereycken, 1983), and this social role may be particularly conducive to the development of the problem (cf. Foa *et al.*, 1984). One view of the disorder suggests that the person feels trapped in an unsatisfactory relationship because of a fear of leaving and living independently (Goldstein & Chambless, 1978). This is consistent with formulations of the disorder in terms of unresolved dependency (Weiss, 1964) or anxious attachment (Bowlby, 1969), but evidence of a causal role for marital problems or lack of assertion is poor (Buglass *et al.*, 1977; Foa *et al.*, 1984; Vandereycken, 1983). Interpersonal difficulties are often produced by the problem itself (Burns & Thorpe, 1977), and may be alleviated by its improvement (Cobb, McDonald, Marks & Stern, 1980). Close relationships also form an important predictor of treatment success. Exposure treatments are less effective, particularly in the long term, if the marital relationship is unsatisfactory (Vandereycken, 1983). A link with sexual dysfunctions was observed in some early studies (e.g. Webster, 1953), although more recent observations have shown a lower incidence and suggest that often these dysfunctions are consequences of the agoraphobia (Buglass *et al.*, 1977; Foa *et al.*, 1984).

Social phobia and simple phobia

Other phobias are often divided into social phobias (DSM-III-R, American Psychiatric Association, 1987). In *social* phobias, the fear and avoidance is focused on situations in which the person performs an activity under the possible scrutiny of others, such as eating, signing a form or speaking in public. Specific or *simple* phobias involve other situations or objects, such as dogs, heights and closed spaces. The identification of social phobias as a separate group draws attention to the concern over social humiliation and embarrassment, although this concern can also emerge in relation to agoraphobia or other specific fears. Social phobias are probably better seen as a subgroup of specific phobias. Names of some simple phobias are shown in Table 2.1.

Multiple specific phobias or 'mixed' phobias may occur. Often an individual will seek treatment for one of these phobias, and only on specific questioning will further fears be revealed. Although these may be completely unrelated, sometimes themes will emerge that assist in ascertaining the precise elements in each specific phobia. For example, a fear of elevators and other small rooms suggests a different dimension of the situation than a fear of elevators and high places.

Table 2.1: *Names for selected specific phobias*

acrophobia	heights
ailurophobia	cats
arachnophobia	spiders
avisophobia	birds
brontophobia	storms
cancerophobia	cancer
claustrophibia	closed spaces
cynophobia	dogs
hippophobia	horses
insectophobia	insects
mysophobia	dirt
nosophobia	illness/injury
nyctophobia	darkness
ophidiophobia	snakes
rodentophobia	rodents
thanatophobia	death
venerophobia	sexually-transmitted disease

For both social and simple phobias, DSM-III-R (American Psychiatric Association, 1987), demands that: (a) during some phase of the problem, exposure to the specific phobic stimulus almost invariably provoked an immediate anxiety response, and that (b) the object or situation is avoided or endured with intense anxiety. It distinguishes phobic disorders from more commonplace fears by restricting the classification to situations when (c) the avoidance behaviour or fear causes marked distress or interferes with social or occupational functioning. To exclude adaptive responses to dangerous situations, it also requires that (d) there is recognition by the individual that his or her fear is excessive or unreasonable. The phobic stimulus must also be unrelated to other co-existing disorders.

Generalised anxiety

This chapter has not invoked traditional distinctions between fear and anxiety, either in terms of the degree of objective danger or the specific stimulus focus of the cognitions that accompany the fear. Whether there is a cognitive focus for the emotion does not demonstrably change the emotional response itself, and it often represents a tentative hypothesis regarding the fear or anxiety that is only advanced after the emotion is experienced. This is especially likely in panic disorder and agoraphobia, where the fear often appears diffuse and unrelated to stimulus conditions, even when there is an objectively verifiable relationship.

The emotion of fear or anxiety can also appear as a persistent state that is widely generalised across situations, but is not accompanied by agoraphobic avoidance or punctuated by discrete panic attacks. Generalised anxiety disorder (GAD) in DSM-III-R (American Psychiatric Association, 1987) requires that the person has been 'bothered more days than not' by 'unrealistic and excessive worry (apprehensive expectation) about two or more life circumstances' over a period of at least six months. He or she must also show 6 out of 18 anxiety features that involve motor tension, autonomic hyperactivity or vigilance and scanning. To reduce confusion with other categories, the focus of the worry must be unrelated to any co-existing mental disorder, it may not occur only during the course of a mood disorder or psychotic disorder, and it cannot be sustained by a known organic factor.

Post-traumatic stress disorder (PTSD)

Sometimes individuals have experienced an event that is unusual and psychologically highly traumatic, such as witnessing extreme physical violence or being under serious physical threat. These people frequently experience effects of this experience that may persist for many years (Archibald & Tuddenham, 1965). DSM-III-R (American Psychiatric Association, 1987) requires that three types of problems all occurred persistently during at least one month. These are: (a) cognitive or affective re-experiencing of the event; (b) avoidance of associated stimuli (or a numbing of affective responsiveness); and (c) symptoms of increased physiological arousal that were not present before the trauma.

Similar features may, of course, be seen during the development of many phobias, and chronic phobic reactions are often the vestiges of a traumatic experience. Separation of the more spectacular traumas into PTSD may assist the person to avoid the opprobrium that often accompanies other psychiatric diagnoses, but would do little to further a scientific study of behavioural disorders if the difference were merely one of degree. In fact, there is considerably more to PTSD, which is frequently associated with problems such as depression and anger as well as anxiety. The DSM categorisation of PTSD under anxiety disorders remains a somewhat poor reflection of the complex family of PTSD disorders that are encountered in clinical practice. A review of assessment issues in combat-related PTSD is provided by Wolfe, Keene, Lyons & Geraldi (1987).

The interview

Although the above description of anxiety disorders is closely linked to DSM-III-R categories, the interview below is not intended primarily as an instrument for diagnosis. Other structured interviews such as 'The structured clinical interview for DSM-III-R' (SCID; Spitzer, Williams & Gibbon, 1987) are available for this purpose. Instead, it aims at a functional analysis of the person's problems, whether or not they fulfil the formal criteria for DSM-III-R. For example, the present chapter includes consideration of fears that do not meet criteria for phobias, because clients may often request treatment for other fears. A man who is afraid of surgery may not see his fear as unreasonable or excessive, but may still require assistance in dealing with his problem. The functional analysis of this fear and the use of a behavioural treatment is not compromised by its failure to meet DSM-III-R criteria.

As discussed in the introductory chapter, the assessment interview should begin with the client giving an account of the problem in his/her own words. This will alert the interviewer to particular aspects that should be emphasised in the remainder of the interview. The following questions can be reworded or reordered to reflect these emphases. They assume that the interviewer already has obtained biographical information from the client (see Chapter 1).

Last occasion

When was the last time that you experienced the problem? What happened?

After the person has described the event in his own words, complete the description with questions such as:

What sorts of physical sensations did you have? Do you remember what you were thinking of? What did you do? What happened afterwards?

Was that a typical example? *If not:* In what way did it differ?

Frequency and antecedents

How often does the problem occur?

Are there any situations where the problem is worse, or occurs more frequently *or* any that you always avoid or have difficulty coping with?

If yes:

What is the very worst you can imagine? What situations are easier to confront? What makes these situations easier?

Are there any other things that provoke anxiety?

These questions allow a preliminary assessment of situational dimensions. Individuals may regard situations as easier to confront when they expect them to be more predictable, to require a lower degree of performance skills, or to result in less negative consequences if they fail to deal with them effectively. Examples of this are when the interaction is time-limited, when the feared object is restrained or at a further distance and when assistance such as equipment or other people are available (cf Bandura, 1982). Common dimensions in agoraphobia were discussed above. Notice non-phobic aspects that may trigger panic attacks such as hot weather or exercise.

Physical reactions

What physical reactions do you usually have?

After the person has described these without prompting:

Are you ever short of breath or do you ever have difficulty breathing? Do you have any chest pain or discomfort? Do you notice your heart beating quickly, or do you have any palpitations? Do you have any sweating, or hot or cold flashes? Do you feel dizzy or about to faint? Do you experience any nausea or internal discomfort or numbness or tingling sensations or any trembling or shaking?

How often do you have these feelings?

Do they start suddenly, or build up slowly?

When do you start to notice them?

What is happening then?

When are they at their worst?

How long do they last?

Behaviour

What do you do when you think you might encounter the situation or have an anxiety attack?

If the situation (or attack) does occur, what do you do then?

Look for: (a) methods used to avoid the situation or escape from it; (b) coping behaviours such as relaxation or meditation, or attempts to make the situation more predictable; (c) the use of food, alcohol, prescribed or illegal drugs to reduce discomfort. Note that the severity of the problem may not affect the overall effectiveness of a participant treatment, but may necessitate the greater use of performance aids (Bandura, Jeffrey & Wright, 1974).

Cognitions

How often do you worry about the problem? What do you think about?
What thoughts or images do you have when you are about to be faced with the situation or when you think that an anxiety attack is coming?
What images or thoughts go through your mind when it is happening?
After it is over, what do you think about then?

Look for either cognitions that assist and undermine successful coping with the situation. Important types of cognitions include self-efficacy, or self-judged capability to perform coping behaviours, beliefs about the danger of the situation or irrationality of the fear and avoidance, and beliefs about the meaning or effects of physical sensations, especially concerning panic attacks (e.g. concern that they herald a terminal illness or madness, or concern over losing control in public). These cognitions need not be verbal, e.g. they may be experienced as images of inadequate coping or of a disastrous outcome. Cognitive/perceptual responses to an anxiety reaction may also include depersonalisation, where there is a sense of observing oneself perform rather than deliberately acting, and derealisation, where the person's voice may sound strange or the surroundings may appear vague or unstable. If the anxiety arises from a traumatic experience, the person may have vivid recollections of the event.

History

How long has the fear or avoidance been occurring?

Phobics often experienced fears in childhood (Ollendick, 1979), and retrospective reports suggest that specific animal fears in adulthood frequently originate before the age of five (Marks & Gelder, 1966). Agoraphobics, whose problem typically begins in early adulthood, become disabled in about 15 months but do not seek help for an average of 13 years (Marks & Herst, 1970). The fact that a client has not sought treatment for a long-standing fear does not necessarily mean that the fear or avoidance is of mild intensity or is easier to treat. In fact, if the fear and avoidance have become a stable feature of the person's life, both the client and significant others may initially be sceptical of the chance for improvement, and the behavioural adjustments may be well entrenched.

How did the problem start?

Was anything else happening to you at the time?

These questions can assist in developing hypotheses concerning the parameters of current fear and avoidance, and about stressful contextual factors.

Fluctuating severity

Have there been periods when you have been more able to cope with the situation? When was the last time? What was happening then?

Note illnesses, menstrual cycles, anniversaries, changes in interpersonal circumstances. For example, agoraphobia tends to have a fluctuating course. One-third of the sample in Buglass *et al.* (1977) ranged from being completely housebound to no avoidance over a month. However, for most phobics the problem is never completely absent.

Consequences

What effects does the problem have on your life?

Search for both negative consequences and positive effects such as being able to avoid unpleasant tasks.

How do you deal with the restrictions that the problem imposes?

Interpersonal aspects

What effects does the problem have on other people?

How do they feel about that?

Twenty per cent of the agoraphobia sample in Burns & Thorpe (1977) said the agoraphobia was a strain on their marriage. This may often be alleviated by treatment of the fear and avoidance (Cobb *et al.*, 1980). Investigate how satisfactory and rewarding marital and other close relationships are. Problems unrelated to the fear and avoidance may or may not be assisted by treatment and are likely to impede maintenance of improvement (Vandereycken, 1983).

What does your best friend think the problem is?

What does your spouse or partner think about it?

How do other people think you should deal with it?

Conceptions of the problem and its treatment that differ markedly from the therapist's can produce problems later, e.g. when other people fail to reward attempts at coping. A joint consultation explaining the rationale for the treatment strategy may be required.

Current motivation for treatment

Why have you come for treatment now?
Has the problem become worse lately?
Are there any recent changes in other people's reactions?

Previous treatment

Have you seen anyone else about the fear, or about any other psychological problem?
When? Did the treatment work? Is it continuing? *If not:* Why?
Previous experiences may colour the client's motivation to engage in present treatment, and concurrent treatments may conflict with the one proposed.

Physical investigations

Particularly for panic reactions:
Have you had a physical checkup recently?
If yes:
What was the result? Did you discuss your anxiety attacks?
Do you drink coffee or tea?
Intake of caffeine about one gram per day (about 8–10 cups of coffee or 15 cups of tea) may precipitate anxiety reactions (DSM-III-R, American Psychiatric Association, 1987; Veleber & Templer, 1984).
Do you take any tablets? or drink alcohol? or take any other drugs?
Panic-like symptoms can come from intoxication with a stimulant, or withdrawal from a depressant drug. Note also that many people who have anxiety problems try to control their symptoms by self-medicating with depressant drugs (Bibb & Chambless, 1986). Refer to Chapter 9 for further assessment of substance abuse if necessary.

Other problems

It is important to differentiate phobic and anxiety problems from schizophrenic or schizoid disorders. This may be especially significant for some cases of social anxiety or phobia, where difficulties in sustaining close relationships and paranoid feelings may not immediately be detected. Early phases of schizophrenic episodes may also mimic other anxiety disorders. Note that phobic and anxiety reactions also frequently appear in obsessive–compulsive problems and that anxiety is a common secondary feature of a major depressive episode. Even after people who fulfil criteria for 'major depressive episode' are excluded, about half of agoraphobics report dysphoric mood (Buglass *et al.*, 1977; Foa *et al.*, 1984). It is likely that depression may assist in the development of maintenance of agoraphobia (e.g. through depressive withdrawal and perceived inefficacy), and that agoraphobic withdrawal and inefficacy exacerbates depression (cf Foa *et al.*, 1984). Often anxiety reactions are also implicated in a range of other problems such as insomnia and sexual dysfunction, and insomnia and/or depression may also be encountered in PTSD (Wolfe *et al.*, 1987). Screening assessments for all of these conditions are therefore recommended.

Specific assessment measures

Self-report measures of general anxiety

Perhaps the best-known scale of general anxiety is the 'Taylor manifest anxiety scale' (MAS; Taylor, 1953) which has been used extensively in research as a measure of trait anxiety. For clinical applications, the 'State–trait anxiety inventory, form Y' (STAI; Speilberger, Gorusch, Lushene, Vagg & Jacobs, 1983) has greater utility, since it provides a reliable and valid index of the immediate anxiety state as well as trait anxiety. To deal with problems of self-disclosure, the 'IPAT anxiety scale questionnaire' (ASQ; Krug, Scheier & Cattell, 1976) derives measures of both overt and covert trait anxiety by using some items that have high statistical but low-content validity. The 'Self-rating anxiety scale' (SAS; Zung & Cavenar, 1980) allows the clinician to sample 5 affective and 15 somatic symptoms of anxiety. Finally, Lehrer & Woolfolk (1982) present an anxiety scale that provides separate scores relating to somatic, cognitive and behavioural reactions relating to fear and anxiety. Structured interviews for anxiety disorders include the 'Hamilton anxiety scale' (Hamilton, 1959) and the 'Anxiety disorders interview' (DiNardo, O'Brien, Barlow, Waddell & Blanchard, 1983).

Trait anxiety has a close relationship with the emotionality or neuroticism factor in the 'Eysenck personality scales' — the 'Eysenck personality inventory' (EPI; Eysenck & Eysenck, 1964) and the 'Eysenck personality questionnaire' (EPQ; Eysenck & Eysenck, 1975). For example, the correlation between the ASQ and EPI-N scale is 0.79 (Krug *et al.*, 1976). While general measures of anxiety and neuroticism can be used to obtain an overall index, they suffer from the problem of low correlations with indices of behaviour in specific situations (Mischel, 1968). For more successful predictions, the self-report measures themselves must become specific.

Fear survey measures

Inspired by the *Fear survey schedule–1* (Lang & Lazovik, 1963), a number of screening measures have been developed (e.g. the *FSS–II*, Bernstein & Allen, 1969; Geer, 1965; *FSS–III*, Wolpe & Lang, 1964; and the 'Temple fear survey inventory, Braun & Reynolds, 1969). Each asks for ratings of fear intensity about a number of situations, and there is a substantial item overlap between the scales. The latest version of these scales is the 'Wolpe–Lange augmented FSS' (Wolpe & Lang, 1969), which has 108 items. Fischer & Turner (1978) and Tomlin, Thyer, Curtis, Nesse, Cameron & Wright (1984) have published norms for this measure. Good reliability has typically been found for fear survey schedules, but as with general anxiety questionnaires, they show relatively poor correlations with performance (Hersen, 1973; Taylor & Agras, 1981). Their major use is in providing a more systematic and wide-ranging sample of fears than is typically obtained at interview. More specific questionnaires have focused on: heights (Baker, Cohen & Saunders, 1973), spiders (Lang, Melamed & Hart, 1970; Watts & Sherrock, 1984), social evaluation (Watson & Friend, 1969), and tests (Alpert & Haber, 1960; Osterhouse, 1972; Sarason, 1972, 1978; Spielberger, Gonzalez, Taylor, Algaze & Anton, 1978; Suinn, 1969; Tryon, 1980). The 'mobility inventory for agoraphobia' was presented by Chambless, Caputo, Jasin, Gracely & Williams (1985). This asks about avoidance of situations when alone and when accompanied by another person. It also assesses the frequency of panic attacks over the previous 7 days. Preliminary data on the scale are encouraging. Marks & Mathews (1979) also attempted a compromise between a broad and highly specific measure. Subjects rate their mood and judge the degree to which they avoid 16 commonly feared situations and also report their avoidance of their main phobic situation. However, S. Williams & Rappoport (1983) found that even this specific rating failed to correlate with a behavioural test of driving alone, and that it overestimated the true impact of treatment.

Concurrent fear and avoidance measures

Concurrent ratings of fear during a performance attempt can be made on the 'fear thermometer' of Walk (1956) which has a scale from 0–10, or the Wolpe (1969) 'subjective units of distress scale' (SUDS). On the SUDS scale, 0 is described as absolute calm and 100 is the worst anxiety ever experienced, or the worst the person can imagine feeling. Significant relationships between SUDS scores and hand temperature were observed in Thyer, Papsdorf, Davis & Vallecorsa (1984).

Examples of *self-monitoring* forms are provided in Tables 2.2, 2.3 and 2.4. Table 2.2 is an anxiety-monitoring form that will assist in identifying the critical situations and cognitions in causes of diffuse anxiety. It also elicits activities and cognitions that can potentially be used as coping strategies. Table 2.3 shows a form for monitoring events that the individual finds anxiety-provoking. Thoughts, coping behaviours and consequences are also recorded. The form in Table 2.4 is designed for monitoring panic attacks. Clients are given only one of these forms at any time, and the retention of the same anxiety scale allows some comparability across forms. Note that clients will often require training in becoming aware of cognitions that occur in the fear or anxiety situations. Some idea of these can be obtained at the initial interview, and questioning at the end of the first week of monitoring can provide a further prompt. When recording encounters with feared situations, clients should be reminded to record actions that effectively prevent the situation from occurring, e.g. a snake phobic is likely to place a standing veto on family outings to forest settings. Even so, this form by itself is likely to underestimate the restrictions imposed on the life of a person with a well-established phobia.

Psychophysiological measures will not be reviewed here. Issues of measurements are discussed in Sturgis & Arena (1984), Arena, Blanchard, Andrasik, Cotch & Myers (1983), and Taylor & Agras (1981). These measures often show relatively low concordance with behaviour and self-reported fear (Kaloupek & Levis, 1983; Lang, 1968, 1971).

Table 2.2: *Anxiety-monitoring form*

Each rating of anxiety is made on a scale, using numbers to indicate how you felt.

0	2	4	6	8	10
No anxiety at all		Moderately anxious			Extremely anxious. The worst I can imagine feeling

Day ____________ Date ____________

Please circle the number (from 0 to 10) which indicates how you felt today.

(A) When you felt the BEST: Time of day ____________
Rating 0 2 4 6 8 10
What were you doing?
What were you thinking?

(B) *When you felt WORST*: Time of day ____________
Rating 0 2 4 6 8 10
What were you doing?
What were you thinking?

Day ____________ Date ____________

Please circle the number (from 0 to 10) which indicates how you felt today.

(A) *When you felt the BEST*: Time of day ____________
Rating 0 2 4 6 8 10
What were you doing?
What were you thinking?

(B) *When you felt WORST*: Time of day ____________
Rating 0 2 4 6 8 10
What were you doing?
What were you thinking?

Measurement of self-efficacy

Self-efficacy measures typically list situations or tasks in hierarchical order and ask clients to designate whether they can perform each task right now. For each task clients check, they rate the strength of their expectations on a 100-point probability scale that ranges in 10-unit intervals, from quite uncertain to certain. An example is in Table 2.5, which is adapted from Kavanagh, Knight & Ponzio (1986). Tasks in the hierarchy should lend themselves to behaviour observation and be sufficiently close in

Table 2.3: *Monitoring form for encounters with feared situations*

Please record any times when you thought you might encounter the objects or situations that worry you, i.e.

....

....

Describe:
* the time and place
* the situation
* what you thought
* what you did
* what happened then
* maximum anxiety during the experience on the following scale:

0	2	4	6	8	10
No anxiety at all		Moderately anxious			Extremely anxious. The worst I can imagine feeling

Date:	Situation:						
Time:	Thought:						
Place:	Did:						
....	Then:						
	Maximum anxiety:	0	2	4	6	8	10
Date:	Situation:						
Time:	Thought:						
Place:	Did:						
....	Then:						
	Maximum anxiety:	0	2	4	6	8	10
Date:	Situation:						
Time:	Thought:						
Place:	Did:						
....	Then:						
	Maximum anxiety:	0	2	4	6	8	10
Date:	Situation:						
Time:	Thought:						
Place:	Did:						
....	Then:						
	Maximum anxiety:	0	2	4	6	8	10

Table 2.4: *Monitoring form for panic attacks*

A panic attack is a rush of anxiety and intense physical reactions that reach a peak within about 10 minutes. Please record any panic attacks that you experience.

Describe: * *when* the attack *began* and *ended*
* *the situation* (Where were you? What was happening? Who was there?)
* your *physical reactions*
* what you *thought*
* what you *did* to cope with the attack
* what happened *then*
* your *maximum anxiety* during the attack, on the following scale:

0	2	4	6	8	10
No anxiety at all		Moderately anxious			Extremely anxious. The worst I can imagine feeling

Date:......................	Situation: ....
Time began.............	Physical reactions: ....
Time ended:............	Thought: ....
Maximum anxiety:	Did:..
0 2 4 6 8 10	Then:..
Date:......................	Situation: ....
Time began.............	Physical reactions: ....
Time ended:............	Thought: ....
Maximum anxiety:	Did:..
0 2 4 6 8 10	Then:..
Date:......................	Situation: ....
Time began.............	Physical reactions: ....
Time ended:............	Thought: ....
Maximum anxiety:	Did:..
0 2 4 6 8 10	Then:..

difficulty that they are sensitive to intermediate changes in efficacy and performance. Individualised scales will often therefore be needed for particular clients. To maximise their predictive power, the measures are normally given immediately prior to performance. The self-efficacy level is the maximum task clients think they can accomplish. Strength of self-efficacy is measured by

Table 2.5: *Example of self-efficacy scale*

The following items are about having needles. Under the *Can Do* column, check (√) the items you expect you could do if you were asked to do them now.

For the items you check under *Can Do*, indicate in the *Confidence* column how confident you are that you could do them. Rate your degree of confidence by recording a number from 10 to 100 using the scale given below:

10	20	30	40	50	60	70	80	90	100
quite uncertain				moderately certain					certain

Remember, rate what you expect you could do and your confidence if you were asked to perform the tasks *now*.

Tasks	*Can do*	*Confidence*
Leave for clinic	______	______
Enter clinic	______	______
Wait for doctor	______	______
Sit through preliminary discussion	______	______
Sit through needle preparation	______	______
Stay for skin swabs and needle positioning	______	______
Have a subcutaneous injection (25 gauge)	______	______
Have an intramuscular injection (25 gauge)	______	______
Have an intravenous injection (21 gauge)	______	______
Blood sample while seated, therapist present	______	______
Blood sample while seated, therapist absent	______	______
Blood sample lying down, therapist absent	______	______

taking the average strength rating over the total number of tasks.

Correlations of level and strength of self-efficacy with subsequent performance range as high as 0.70 or more (Bandura, 1977b). The self-efficacy scale also allows a task-by-task analysis of the match between expectation and performance. This microanalytic strategy yields a measure of percentage congruence that often reaches 80 to 90 per cent (Bandura, 1977b, 1982; Cervone, 1985). Self-efficacy ratings may even exceed past performance as a predictor of later performance, especially when significant change in the situation has occurred (Bandura, 1982). Since self-efficacy is such a strong predictor of performance, its assessment is highly recommended.

Forming a hierarchy

Using information about dimensions of feared situations that was gained at the first interview, the therapist generates a series of tasks that can form a treatment hierarchy. For *in vivo* treatment, these tasks should obviously be ones that are easily administered, but should maximise generalisation to the troublesome situations the client will encounter outside treatment. So, for example, an agoraphobic who has trouble with supermarket queues should be trained in that situation where possible, but pragmatic considerations may demand that the supermarket be within travelling distance of both therapist and client. Once a menu of possible tasks has been generated, the client is traditionally asked to rate each of these tasks on a fear thermometer (Walk, 1956) or in SUDS units (Wolpe, 1969; see p. 37). These ratings are used to select items that will form a hierarchy of expected fear. Large steps between the difficulty of succeeding items are filled by new items where necessary.

The rating of the hierarchy in terms of fear value harks back to the centrality of the anxiety within two-factor theory and the treatment format of systematic desensitisation. If pride of place were to be seceded to self-efficacy about dealing with the situation (Bandura, 1986), presumably the hierarchy should be in terms of self-efficacy or of perceived difficulty rather than fear or anxiety.

Measurement of behaviour

People who report excessive fears and regular avoidance of the phobic stimulus often show little behavioural avoidance when this is tested at initial assessment (e.g. Lang, 1968; Williams & Rappoport, 1983). For this reason, reports of unusual performance should be supplemented with behaviour observations that are standardised across time for the individual client. Behavioural approach tests (BAT) within the laboratory were pioneered by Lang & Lazovik (1963). The person was asked to approach a snake as close as possible and if possible, to handle it. Similar hierarchical tasks have been used with a number of fears (Taylor & Agras, 1981). Their major weakness is their likely vulnerability to situational specificity (Mischel, 1968). In particular, the incentives for approach and assurance of ultimate protection are probably much greater than in the natural environment. Their value as indicators of usual behaviour is therefore limited by these differences. In order to reduce this problem, recent studies have often used behavioural tests where clients attempted the tasks alone and in natural settings (e.g. Ost, Jerremalm & Jansson, 1984; Williams & Rappoport, 1983), perhaps even monitoring their own behaviour between sessions (e.g. Mathews, Teasdale, Munby, Johnston & Shaw, 1977). Hierarchies formed by methods described in the previous section can be used as the basis for behavioural tests in the laboratory or in naturalistic settings.

Behavioural manifestations of anxiety can also be measured during a performance attempt. For example, the 'timed behaviour checklist' of Paul (1966) listed 20 behaviours such as pacing, swaying, speech blocks or stammers, which were checked during successive 30-second intervals of a speech presentation. Paul was able to obtain an average interrater reliability of over 0.95 after training.

Treatment of anxiety disorders

Recent interviews of treatment procedures are given by Rimm & Lefebvre (1981) for phobias generally, and by Mathews, Gelder & Johnston (1981) for agoraphobia. Treatments for specific anxiety disorders are also reviewed in Turner (1984), and treatment manuals are provided by Mathews *et al.* (1981) and Barlow (1985). Approaches to PTSD are discussed in Fairbank & Brown (1987). Specific treatments for anxiety and fear include:

1. *Participant modelling and other in vivo procedures.* The combination of modelling with *in vivo* participation appears to be a particularly powerful treatment for specific phobias (Bandura *et al.*, 1969; Bandura *et al.*, 1974; Etringer, Cash & Rimm, 1982). *In vivo* treatments were reviewed by Linden (1981). Note that for agoraphobia, the primary situational focus for *in vivo* treatment may be the hyperventilation or panic experience (Grattan, Wilson & Franklin, 1987).

2. *Relaxation training and biofeedback.* A standard relaxation training manual is given by Bernstein & Borkovec (1973). Reviews include Glaister (1982), Hillenberg & Collins (1982) and King (1980). The efficacy of biofeedback is reviewed by Rice & Blanchard (1982).
3. *Imaginal systematic desensitisation.* First developed by Wolpe (1958), this procedure is supported by a substantial body of evidence (McGlynn, Mealiea & Landau, 1981) and continues to be widely used. There is some evidence that participant modelling and other *in vivo* procedures are more powerful (Bandura *et al.*, 1969; Linden, 1981).
4. *Cognitive treatments* for anxiety and stress have been advanced by Beck & Emery (1979) and Meichenbaum (1977). These were reviewed by Last (1984). At this stage, there is little evidence that cognitive techniques contribute additional strength to *in vivo* procedures for phobias (Williams & Rappoport, 1983), although they are likely to be very important in treatment of worry.

3
Depression

Introduction

Problems involving depressed mood are amongst the most common psychological complaints both in the general community and in the clinical population. About 20 per cent of people experience significant depression at some point in their lives, although the inclusion of milder forms of depressed mood would increase this proportion considerably. While common usage of the word 'depression' refers to general feeling of unhappiness and sadness, the term is also used in a clinical sense to refer to a collection of signs and symptoms that constitute a syndrome. There are several diagnostic categories in DSM-III-R (American Psychiatric Association, 1987) in which depressive features may form a major part of the clinical picture. The most important of these categories is 'major depressive episode', which requires the presence of at least five of the following symptoms nearly every day for a period of at least two weeks, including one or other of the first two symptoms listed: (1) dysphoric mood; (2) loss of interest or pleasure in all (or almost all) usual activities; (3) decreased appetite or weight loss (or increased appetite and weight gain); (4) insomnia or hypersomnia; (5) psychomotor retardation or agitation; (6) loss of energy or feelings of fatigue; (7) feelings of worthlessness, or excessive or inappropriate guilt; (8) diminished ability to think, concentrate, make decisions; and (9) recurrent thoughts of death, or suicidal thoughts or actions. (The manual should be consulted for certain exclusion criteria.)

A major depressive episode, often referred to as unipolar depression, needs to be clearly distinguished from disorders involving alternation between depressive and manic periods, a condition generally referred to as 'bipolar affective disorder' or 'manic depressive disorder'. The criteria for manic episode in DSM-III-R include prominent elevated, expansive or irritable mood, in combination with three of the following: (1) inflated self-esteem or grandiosity; (2) decreased need for sleep; (3) more talkative than usual; (4) flight of ideas or racing thoughts; (5) distractability; (6) increased activity or psychomotor agitation; and (7) involvement in activities without consideration of consequences (e.g. spending large amounts of money, sexual indiscretions). (Please check the manual for certain exclusion criteria; note also, that four of the accompanying symptoms need to be present if the mood is only irritable, without being elevated or expansive.) These criteria are mentioned here primarily because the clinician needs to be aware that manic symptomatology, either alone or in alternation with depressive features, may constitute a disorder of potentially psychotic qualitites characterised by delusions and hallucinations, and will generally require medication and/or hospitalisation during acute episodes. Even an episode of bipolar disorder may commence with a depressive phase, or a mixture of depressive and manic features. Thus, it is important to consider the possible presence of manic symptoms or the previous experience of such features during the course of the initial interview. DSM-III-R also povides for the diagnosis of cyclothymic disorder in cases where there is a chronic (i.e. duration of at least two years) alternation between states of depressive and manic features with less impairment of the person in carrying out normal functions.

Two further DSM-III-R categories in which depressive symptoms predominate are dysthymia and 'adjustment disorder with depression'. Dysthymia involves the presence of at least mild depressive symptoms fairly continuously over a period of at least two years. Dysthymia may also be secondary to another disorder such as anorexia nervosa, substance dependence or anxiety disorder. Adjustment disorder with depression involves an excessive reaction to a psychosocial stressor that has occurred within the three months prior to onset. Symptoms predominantly include depressed mood, tearfulness and feelings of hopelessness. The diagnosis is restricted to episodes of less than six months' duration, and is not part of a previous pattern of overreactions to stress.

As can be seen from the features of 'major depressive episode', this category consists of individuals with a varied set of behavioural, cognitive and somatic symptoms. The heterogeneity of the persons who receive the diagnosis of major depressive episode is evident from the fact that only five of the nine symptoms listed above are required to be present. Dysthymic disorder is also worthy of some attention, because such individuals may frequently seek therapy, either for their chronic depressive features or for other coexistent problems. Some individuals appear to experience a major depressive episode superimposed on a dysthymic disorder, a condition referred to by Keller, Shapiro, Lavori & Wolf (1982) as 'double depression'. Depressive symptoms may also be secondary to other major difficulties, e.g. alcohol abuse, sexual problems, phobias or physical disorders. Thus, the assessment of depression needs to be fairly broad, covering the presenting symptomatology, the time course of such symptoms, general history, other potentially important coexisting psychological complaints and the identification of likely causal factors. In particular, depressive patients may also present with significant levels of generalised or phobic anxiety. Other common concurrent problems include agoraphobia, obsessive–compulsive disorders, social behaviour problems, chronic pain and insomnia. Whether or not all the distinctions between types of affective disorders that are made within DSM-III-R are truly representative of different disorders of separate aetiology remains uncertain. Rather more conviction can be placed in the importance of the distinction between unipolar and bipolar disorders (Depue & Monroe, 1978) than between the suggested unipolar types such as major depressive episode versus dysthymia. Some of the temporal requirements for the presence of disorders, such as a two-week period for major depressive disorder, remain rather arbitrary, as are the prescriptions for a set number of symptoms irrespective of the differential severity of such symptoms. Nevertheless, the DSM system has contributed to a continuing effort to facilitate the reporting of subject characteristics, and to improve the consistency of screening criteria in research studies. In the long term, such application of consistent criteria may help to refine the possible diagnostic distinctions between affective disorders.

It has been widely believed that depressive disorders may be broadly categorised into two types: depressions caused by alterations in brain biochemistry (endogenous) and those that are caused by environmental factors (non-endogenous, neurotic, reactive). These two allegedly different types of depression are thought to be represented by different symptom classes. It is generally thought that endogenous depressions are characterised by a number of features such as: loss of interest in almost all pleasurable activities, lack of reactivity to pleasurable stimuli, depression worse in the morning, early morning awakening, marked psychomotor retardation or agitation and significant weight loss. These depressions often have a clear episodic pattern with almost complete recovery between episodes. Although there is no suggested aetological assumption in DSM-III-R, a person may be diagnosed as having a major depressive episode with features of melancholia, if symptoms similar to those listed above are present (see the DSM-III-R manual for precise details).

Whether or not depressions can be subdivided into endogenous and non-endogenous categories has been a continuing source of controversy during most of this century. An alternative school of thought holds that differences alleged to be associated with the endogenous-reactive distinction merely represent a continuum of severity (Kendell, 1976). There are several pieces of evidence that pose difficulties for the endogenous-reactive distinction, such as the finding in some studies that tricyclic antidepressants are somewhat effective with non-endogenous depressions (e.g. Raskin & Crook, 1976), the evidence that endogenous depressions cannot be distinguished from non-endogenous depression in the occurrence of life events prior to onset (e.g. Paykel, Myers, Dienelt, Klerman, Lindenthal & Pepper, 1969) and the failure to find a clear dichotomy between groups of patients based on the symptom features or other characteristics (Young, Scheftner, Klerman, Andreasen & Hirschfield, 1986; Zimmerman, Coryell, Pfhol & Stangl, 1986).

Life events

There is a considerable body of literature supporting a connection between the occurrence of negative life events and depression (e.g. Brown & Harris, 1978). In particular, events involving some kind of loss (e.g. relationship breakups, divorce, death, loss of employment) are very common precipitants (Paykel *et al.*, 1969), although the effects of such life events appear to be partly dependent upon the level of social support received by the person (Cohen & Wills, 1985). It is also apparent that many depressions appear to occur in the absence of any clear environmental precipitant, although these depressions do not necessarily present with the 'endogenous' set of symptoms. It should also be borne in mind that there are difficulties in the interpretation of many of the studies of life events.

For example, failure to detect events may be partly attributable to an inadequate survey of potentially important events or to an insufficient retrospective time period. In addition, there is considerable difficulty in determining whether an event has occurred as a possible cause or as a consequence of depression. Nevertheless, the weight of evidence does suggest a causal role of adverse life events in many cases and investigation of recent life events is an important area of assessment in depression.

Bereavement and post-natal experiences call for special consideration. It is normal for a person to experience grief following the death of a close friend or family member, and the distinction between such reactions and depression is not precise. The clinician should be cautious in the assessment of the suitability of various types of treatment in cases of recent bereavement. The diagnosis of clinical depression is generally made only when there is a prolonged reaction, e.g. after twelve months. In DSM-III, use is made of the term *uncomplicated bereavement* to refer to the existence of a normal grief reaction, in which full depressive symptoms may be displayed, with less feelings of worthlessness or psychomotor retardation. Some symptoms may be altered in form, e.g. guilt may be focused on feelings that the surviving person should also have died. The interested reader might consult a paper by Brasted & Callahan (1984), which provides a useful overview of the psychological literature on grief.

Postnatal (postpartum/puerperal) depression is a further complex area requiring some specialised knowledge and careful assessment. Cutrona (1982) and Hopkins, Marcus & Campbell (1984) describe three different types of postnatal depression: (1) maternity blues, which occur in a large proportion of women between three and eight days after the birth and usually disappear quickly; (2) postnatal depression without psychotic features, which may last from several weeks to many months; and (3) the much less common condition of postnatal depression with psychotic features, such as a refusal to believe that the birth has taken place, or thoughts of harming the baby. Treatment implications may differ, depending on the type of disorder involved, the severity of the problem, medical and psychiatric history and other psychosocial factors. For example, very close monitoring of the condition, perhaps requiring hospitalisation and medication, ought to be considered when there are psychotic features present.

Theories of depression

Several psychological theories have emerged in the search for an explanation of the cause of depression. These theories include: 'learned helplessness' (Seligman, 1975), and its reformulation (Abramson, Seligman & Teasdale, 1978); 'reduced positive reinforcement' (Lewinsohn, 1975) and the 'cognitive theory' (Beck, Rush, Shaw & Emery, 1979). A detailed review of the status of these theories is beyond the scope of the present text, although a brief overview may be helpful in alerting the reader to those aspects of the individual client's environment, behaviour and cognition that may provide a clue to the likely causal factors and may hold implications for treatment.

Lewinsohn (1975), and Lewinsohn, Youngren & Grosscup (1979) suggested that depression may occur as a result of a reduction in response-contingent positive reinforcement. This reduction may occur 'when the probability that the individual's behavior will be followed by reinforcement is low' or 'when the probability that the individual will be reinforced when he does not emit the behavior is high' (Lewinsohn, 1975, p. 31–2). Cognitive features of depression (low self-esteem, guilt, pessimism) are thought to be a result of attributions that the individual makes about his/her feeling of dysphoria. The total amount of response-contingent positive reinforcement received by an individual is considered to be a function of: (1) the number of events that are potentially reinforcing for the person; (2) the number of such potentially reinforcing events that occur; and (3) the extent to which the person possesses the skill (e.g. social skills) that enables him/her to elicit reinforcement from the environment. Lewinsohn's original position has undergone considerable revision (Lewinsohn, Hoberman, Teri & Hautzinger, 1985). The revised theory involves a sequence of causal connections, beginning with the occurrence of a potentially depression-evoking event that is thought to disrupt the person's automatic behaviour patterns, resulting in a reduced rate of positive reinforcement (and/or an elevated rate of aversive experiences). A result of this sequence of events is considered to be an increase in self-awareness, a state in which there is a focus on the self, increased self-criticism and negative expectations, leading to increased dysphoria and various behavioural, cognitive, interpersonal and other consequences. Lewinsohn *et al.* (1985) also delineate a number of vulnerability factors (variables that increase the likelihood of depression) including: being female, aged between 20 and 40, previous history of depression, low coping skills, sensitivity to aversive events, low socioeconomic status, self-consciousness, low threshold for evocation of self-schemata, low self-esteem and having children below the age of seven. Based on the existing literature, several immunity factors (variables that protect against depression) are also identified by Lewinsohn *et al.*, such as: learned resourcefulness (a concept advanced by Rosenbaum, 1980), self-perceived social competence, high frequency of pleasant events and a high level of social support. Lewinsohn *et al.* suggest that these vulnerability and immunity factors may affect various causal connections in the general model. The new theory incorporates a very large amount of existing research data, although several key concepts, such as the causal connection involving an increased self-awareness, which is said to result from earlier steps in the sequence, require further research at this stage.

Seligman (1975) hypothesised that depression occurs when an individual perceives a lack of relationship (contingency) between his/her behaviour and important outcomes (positive or aversive events). He coined the term 'learned helplessness' to describe the state of passivity and other features that characterise the person who is exposed to (or who has an expectation of) non-contingency. In the reformulation, consideration was given to the kinds of attributions that individuals make about the cause of their 'helplessness'. Abramson *et al.* (1978) suggest that such attributions may vary along several dimensions: personal – universal; global – specific; stable – unstable. Thus, a person who attributes failure in an exam to the fact that he/she was intellectually mediocre would be making a personal, stable and global attribution. Whereas, someone who attributed the failure to the fact that the exam wasn't fair would be making a universal, unstable and specific attribution. In general, the more personal, stable and global are the attributions about negative events, the more likely is the person to be depressed and to experience low self-esteem. The opposite pattern of attributions would hold for positive events. Abramson *et al.* also argue that some of the features of depression are determined by the particular types of attributions made by the person, such as the occurrence of low self-esteem as a result of personal attribution. Although the learned helplessness theory has received considerable support in studies of non-depressed subjects who have been exposed to either uncontrollable, controllable or no aversity stimulation (e.g. Miller & Seligman, 1975), the present status of the attributional reformulation remains controversial (Brewin, 1985; Coyne & Gotlib, 1983).

Present empirical work on the causes of depression is largely dominated by the cognitive theory proposed by Beck *et al.* (1979). Beck argues that depression occurs as a result of the negatively distorted cognitive appraisals made by the person about the events and situations they encounter. He suggests that depressive thinking is characterised by specific illogical processes such as arbitrary inference, selective abstraction, overgeneralisation and magnification. He considers that these negative distortions reflect a fundamental problem in schematic processing of information from the environment. Although he does not clearly specify the origin of such distorted schematic processing, it is suggested that it may result from learning through exposure to prior events and situations. Beck's theory has been subjected to a considerable amount of empirical testing that has produced findings consistent with the theory, although the results of many of these experiments could have alternative interpretations. For example, evidence that depressives engage in negative cognitive distortions provides no information about the causal direction. Such thought processes may be a result of depression rather than a cause of the disorder. In addition, some research has produced results that are inconsistent with the theory (e.g. Lewinsohn, Mischel, Chaplin & Barton, 1980). For a review of the status of Beck's cognitive theory and learned helplessness, the reader is encouraged to consult Coyne & Gotlib (1983), and the subsequent interchange between Coyne & Gotlib (1986) and Segal & Shaw (1986a, 1986b). The papers by Power & Champion (1986) and Teasdale (1983) also provide stimulating discussion of the many conceptual issues involved in the cognitive theories of depression.

Another major approach to the understanding of depression has resulted from biochemical research. The most generally accepted biochemical theories suggest that depression is associated with lowered availability of certain neurotransmitters, such as norepinephrine and/or serotonin at receptor sites in the limbic system. There is some suggestion that biochemical subtypes of depression may exist in which depletions of different neurotransmitters are implicated in different individuals. There is considerable evidence to support a neurotransmitter depletion hypothesis, although some specific aspects of the theory remain controversial. A major question that is not addressed by the biochemical theory that concerns the cause of any such biochemical changes. At best, the evidence supports an association between norepinephrine and/or lowered availability of serotonin and depression, but such changes might not necessarily be the primary causal agent. It is possible that some biochemical changes occur as a result of depression, or that changes in biochemistry might also occur as a result of exposure to certain environmental stressors (Weiss, Glazer, Pohorecky, Brick & Miller, 1975; Weiss, Stone & Harrell, 1970). For an overview of the current status of the biochemical theories and their relationship to antidepressant drug treatment, the reader is referred to a recent paper by McNeal & Cimbolic (1986).

The present, albeit brief, review of the theories of depression highlights the lack of consensus about the cause of one of the most common psychological problems. One difficulty that is faced by all the major theories is that of determining the causal connection between the proposed mechanism and the symptomatology of depression. It is also possible that unnecessary confusion exists about the level of explanation being offered. For example, a biochemical hypothesis is not necessarily inconsistent with certain psychological accounts. Most contemporary theorists, such as Depue (1979) or Akiskal & McKinney (1975) emphasise the need for an integration of information coming from studies of stressful events, coping strategies and biochemical activity.

Depression is a multifaceted problem characterised by a large range of features that may or may not be present in any given individual. A major aim of the assessment ought to be directed towards the identification of the specific deficits, positive attributes and problem areas in a particular individual. These areas include: occurrence of recent life events, negatively distorted cognitive appraisal of events and situations, social-skills deficits, changes in receipt of positive reinforcement and exposure to uncontrollable aversive situations. As mentioned previously, various theorists have placed their emphasis on these areas in their formulations of causal processes. However, it is not being argued here that all theories are equally correct, rather, that different theorists have detected potentially important aspects of depression, some of which may have aetiological significance, whilst others may simply be epiphenomena or even consequences of depression. It is possible that at some point in the future, a basic mechanism will be discerned that will have more explanatory power in the aetiology of depression.

The interview

General considerations

From the foregoing, one can see that the assessment of a person who presents with depressive complaints needs to be fairly broad. It may be helpful to have a general guide to the planning of the session prior to the elaboration of the interview itself. The interview will need to establish answers to the following general questions:

1. Does the person present with symptoms consistent with a diagnosis of depression?
2. If 'yes', do these features correspond to a major depressive episode, dysthymic disorder, bipolar affective disorder or other types?
3. What are the likely causal and maintenance factors?
4. What other problems does the person report?

In obtaining answers to these questions, it is clearly necessary to take a detailed history of the person's current and previous experiences with depression, and to obtain information about his/her general life circumstances. In order to determine whether the person meets some set of agreed criteria for depression, the clinician needs to ask specifically about the occurrence of various symptoms. One such set of questions that may be helpful in this regard is set out in the following section. It should be noted that the interview plan that follows is intended to have a wide-ranging focus, and is not simply aimed at the assessment of severity. Specific interview schedules such as the 'schedule for affective disorders and schizophrenia' (SADS; Endicott, Cohen, Nee, Fleiss & Sarantakos, 1981; Endicott & Spitzer, 1978) or the 'diagnostic interview schedule' (DIS; Myers *et al.*, 1984) could be consulted for the purpose of making a diagnosis of depression using standard diagnostic criteria.

Affect

The aim of these questions is to determine the presence of depressed mood. There are several questions that deal with changes in mood over the course of time in order to provide a guide to the depth and variability of dysphoria and its reactivity to environmental changes. One should also be on the alert for unusual swings of mood in the positive direction, since these changes may be indicative of bipolar affective disorder or cyclothymic disorder.

In general, how have you been feeling over the past week or so?
How have you been feeling in the morning when you first wake up?
When do you feel best during the day?
When do you feel worst during the day?
How much change in your mood have you noticed from day to day?
When you are feeling really down, is there anything that can cheer you up?

If 'yes':

If you have been feeling OK, what sorts of things are likely to make you feel down?
Do you have the feeling that your mood is totally independent of anything that happens to you?
How would you describe your mood when you are feeling really down . . . what is it like?

Activity and enjoyment

Activity level is generally lowered during a period of depression, and there is often a decrease in pleasure and satisfaction obtained from activities. These questions are designed to assess the current level of activity and any changes that may have occurred recently.

How did you spend your time last weekend?

Try to have the person go through each day in some detail.

Is that typical of how you spend your time? If not, in what way is it atypical?
Would you like to be doing more (or less)? Why?

For working people:

What sort of work do you do?
Do you enjoy it? Has your enjoyment of work changed recently? Why?
Are you able to accomplish your usual amount of work at present?
What do you do after you finish work?

For non-working people:

What do you do during the day? How did you spend your time yesterday? Was that a typical day? How would a typical day differ?
What do you generally do in the evening?
Are there any activities that you have stopped doing or cut down

lately, but that you used to do more often? Why?
How much enjoyment do you obtain from the things you do?
What sort of things do you like doing the most?
How often do you do these things?
Have you been feeling unusually tired?

If 'yes':

Can you tell me more about that?
Have you noticed any change in your interest in sex?

If 'yes', explore this issue to obtain further details.

Social activity

How much time do you spend with other people?
What do you do, i.e. where do you see them and where do you go?

If working:

Do you go out with people from work?

If 'yes':

What sorts of things do you do? How often?
How much time do you spend with your family?
Do you enjoy this time?
Who are the most important people to you, i.e. people with whom you can confide your personal thoughts and feelings? How often do you see them?
Who do you most like spending your time with? How often do you see them?
Are you happy with the amount of social contact that you have at present?
Has the amount of time that you spend with people changed recently? In what way? Why might this have happened?
What sort of opportunities do you have to meet new people, make new friends?

Discuss circumstances under which this occurs.

How much enjoyment do you obtain from being with other people?
Has this level of enjoyment changed lately?

If 'yes':

How has it changed?
How much time do you spend alone? How do you feel when you are alone?

Self-esteem and other cognitive aspects

The cognitive features include negative views about the self, the future and present or past experiences. These features often will be evident without the need for direct questioning. For example, one should look out for statements reflecting lack of confidence, lack of ability, feelings of worthlessness, pessimism, guilt, etc. Some people may need some prompting in order to establish whether such problems are present and thus the following set of questions should be helpful:

How do you think that other people would describe you?
How would you describe yourself?
How do you feel about yourself? What are the good things?
Are there any things about yourself that you would like to change?

If 'yes':

What sorts of things?
Do you ever feel that you are a burden on other people?

If 'yes':

In what way?
Do you ever feel guilty about anything?

If 'yes':

What sorts of things do you feel guilty about?
How do you feel about the future?

The cognitive behaviour therapist will also be wishing to examine the content of many of the appraisals, attributions and other instances of the person's thought processes. Details of procedures for undertaking this kind of analysis are beyond the scope of the present text but are provided in Beck *et al.* (1979).

Suicide

Appraisal of suicidal risk is an important part of the initial assessment of depression. Features associated with higher risk include: expressions of hopelessness, social isolation, alcohol or drug abuse, previous suicidal attempts, clear plan of action, possession of the means to commit suicide, recent stress and ill health. Thus, the interviewer should examine each of these issues in detail. A sudden improvement in mood, often accompanied by an unusual calmness, is also regarded as a potential warning sign of suicidal intent. The previous set of questions makes a good lead into discussion of this sensitive area. The following questions may provide a helpful line of continuance in an interview context:

Do you ever feel so bad that you feel like harming yourself?

Other wording could be:

Do you ever feel so bad that you feel you would be better off dead? *or* do you ever have fantasies about suicide?

If the answer to this question is positive, it would be necessary to assess the suicidal risk involved. Questions such as the following may be helpful: If 'yes':

When was the last time you had these thoughts?

Find out about the circumstances surrounding this event.

Have you felt this in the last week?

Have you any idea as to how you would commit suicide?

If 'yes', find out details.

What has stopped you from carrying out your plans?

This question can provide a useful point from which to begin counselling the suicidal client.

Have you ever attempted to commit suicide in the past?

If 'yes':

When was this?

Can you tell me what led up to this point?

Find out all the relevant details, such as the mode of attempt, reasons for not completing the suicide, results of the attempt, etc. Apart from immediate counselling, the steps that should be taken to reduce the risk of suicide will vary considerably depending upon the circumstances. One should consider the possibility of admission to hospital, the involvement of relatives or significant others or the making of an agreement about future contact at a specific point in time.

Sleep

Sleep difficulties may form a part of the depressive syndrome, but may also occur separately. Thus, it is particularly helpful to ascertain whether the sleep problems predate the depressive disorder. It is also necessary to rule out the possibility that some depressive features such as tiredness and fatigue, decreased enjoyment, etc. are not simply a result of a sleep problem. Note that some depressives actually report sleeping longer than usual (hypersomnia).

How have you been sleeping lately?

Have you had difficulty falling asleep?

How long does it take you to fall asleep on an average night?

Have you had periods when you have woken up in the middle of the night or early in the morning?

Find out details, such as how long the person stays awake, how often, how long this problem has been occurring, etc. Refer to Chapter 7 on insomnia.

How many hours sleep do you have on average?

How do you generally feel in the morning?
How long do you stay in bed before getting up as a rule?
Do you ever decide just not to get up at all? How often? Why?
Do you get dressed or do you often stay in nightwear for some period of the day?
Do you ever go back to bed during the day? How often? When? For how long?

Appetite/weight

Loss of appetite and consequent weight loss is more likely to be present in more severe depressions. One should keep in mind the need to ascertain whether the weight loss is part of the depressive problem, a result of being on a diet, a result of medical illness or an expression of anorexia nervosa. It should also be noted that some people actually eat more and put on weight during periods of depression. Note also that increased weight may be a side effect of some anti-depressant medications. The clinician could examine appetite and weight issues with the following questions:

How has your appetite been lately? (Has it changed?)
Have you noticed any change in your enjoyment of food? In what way?
Have you noticed any change in your weight over the last few weeks or so? In what way?

You may need to follow this material up with further questions concerning their present weight, previous weight, pattern of weight loss over time, relation to the onset of depression, etc.

History

The aim of this section is to obtain a detailed history of the person's experience with depression. Other aspects of the person's general history will also be important, and guidelines for that broader area are presented in Chapter 1. An important aspect of the person's experience of depression concerns the duration and episodicity of the symptoms, since this information will be helpful in determining whether the person displays features of dysthymic disorder, or whether there are discrete episodes of depression, or both. Such information can, in turn, lead to the investigation of different causes of the depression.

How long would you say that you have been feeling like you do now?
Has that been fairly continuous, or have there been periods when things have been better/worse?

Find out more specific details of variation over time.

When did you first start to notice being troubled by feelings of depression?

Do your depressive feelings ever go away for some time, say days/or weeks/or months/or years?

How do you feel when the depression goes away altogether?

How does a period of depression start — is it sudden or is there a slow build-up of feelings?

Does the depression come out of nowhere or do you think that there is there a link with other things which are happening to you? What sort of things?

Why do you think that you get depressed?

Have any things happened to you lately that might be important to mention here?

There may still be only a limited amount of information that comes out of the answer to this last question. In many cases, it is worthwhile to ask explicitly whether certain events have occurred, such as: deaths of close friends or relatives, illnesses in close friends or relatives, relationship break-ups, separations, changed work conditions, changed financial circumstances, disappointments or setbacks, etc.

Do you ever have periods when you feel unusually high or active? Can you describe that for me?

Here, one should check for the presence of manic features.

For women patients:

Are you taking the contraceptive pill?

If 'yes', obtain details of duration, type and effect on mood if possible. Check also on menopause and effects of menstrual periods. See DSM-III-R (Appendix A) for a discussion of pre-menstrual depressive disorder, referred to as late luteal dysphoric disorder.

Antecedents

The main aim of this section is to identify any situations or events that commonly result in feelings of depressive mood. The isolation of such discrete depression-eliciting occasions may be particularly helpful in identifying maladaptive cognitions or ineffective coping skills, that may become the subject of future therapeutic endeavours.

Are there any particular things that, when they happen to you, make you feel depressed?

If 'yes':

What kinds of things are these?
Can you tell me more about these situations?
In the last week or so, when do you think that you felt the worst?
What was happening then?

Here, one might explore the circumstances surrounding that period, including any thoughts that the person may be able to recall about that/those event(s).

In the last week or so, when do you think that you felt the best?
What was happening then?

Consequences of depression

Here, one may look for evidence that the depression has either negative or positive consequences on the person's activities, social interaction, lifestyle, etc. Negative effects may be somewhat more obvious, e.g. limitations on work capacity or opportunities for engagement in satisfying social relationships. Depression may also have a negative effect on people in the person's social environment (see Coyne, 1976). It is possible that other people may start to avoid the person who expresses negative views, or is constantly demanding support. Thus, the individual may perceive accurately negative reactions from others, but may make inaccurate attributions about this behaviour. Positive effects may be more subtle, but can include: reduction in demands made by other people, attention and support, coercive marital interactions, etc. While there may be useful clues to such matters that arise in other parts of the interview, the following questions may help to open up this important topic.

How do you think your life would change if you weren't depressed?
Are other people aware of your feelings of depression? Who?
Do you talk about your feelings of depression to others? How often? What do you say?
How do other people react when you are depressed?
What sort of things do you generally talk about when you are with other people?

The reader is also referred to Chapter 5 on the assessment of social competence for further detailed inquiry into this area.

Life events

This area is likely to be the most difficult aspect of the interview(s). As previously noted, there are numerous potential causes of depression, including both psychological and biochemical factors.

In addition, one needs to distinguish between causal, maintenance and consequential factors. For example, life events such as a loss of a job or marital separation, reported by the person as causal factors, may actually have occurred as a consequence of depression or other psychological problems. It is also possible that these events may have increased the severity of the depression. There may be causal and maintenance factors of which the person is unaware. It is often very helpful to draw up a timeline of key events, variations in depressive intensity, etc. Sometimes, the ordinal sequencing can be extremely helpful in suggesting likely causal connections. A review of recent life events may be helpful as a means of identifying possible aetiological factors.

Let's take a moment to review the events of the past year or so. Have there been any important events that have taken place in your life over the last year?

Any events that are mentioned could be followed by a series of questions, such as the following:

Can you tell me what happened in more detail?

What was the cause of . . . (*referring to the event*)?

How did you react to/cope with/deal with . . . (*referring to the event*)?

In case some events have been forgotten, it is useful to go through a short list:

Have there been any difficulties at work?

What about family difficulties?

Have there been any illnesses or deaths amongst friends or family?

Have there been any other difficulties?

History and present circumstances

The exploration of the person's general history and present life circumstances is seen as crucial to the conduct of initial interviews. In the following section, we have provided an outline of the kinds of questions that might be asked to cover such broad areas. Some of the information may have been obtained during the earlier parts of the interview, and, of course, these sections would be omitted at this point. Other questions may not be appropriate under all circumstances. However, the following set of questions should be a helpful guide to the areas of most relevance.

Past and current treatment

Are you currently taking any tablets (medication)?

If 'yes':
  What are you taking?
Obtain details of all medications and dosages.
  Who prescribed these medications?
  How long have you been taking them?
  What medications have you taken for depression previously?
  How did you respond to those?
  Have you received other types of treatment?
If 'yes':
  What sorts of treatment?
Obtain details such as:
  When? For how long? What was the effect?

Specific assessment methods

There are numerous self-report and clinician-rating depression scales presently being employed to assess the severity of depression, including the 'Beck depression inventory', the 'Zung self-rating depression scale' and the 'Hamilton rating scale for depression'.

The Beck depression inventory

The most commonly used self-report scale is the Beck depression inventory (BDI; Beck, Ward, Mendelson, Mock & Erbaugh, 1961). This test consists of 21 items representing different symptoms of depression, each of which is rated on a 4-point scale (scored from 0 to 3) producing a possible range of scores from 0 to 63. Beck suggests the following cut-offs for various levels of severity of depression: no depression (0–9), mild depression (10–16), moderate depression (17–23), severe depression (24+). It should also be noted that the distribution of BDI scores is heavily skewed, thus it is very unusual to find scores above 35. The reader might also consult Kendall, Hollon, Beck, Hammen & Ingram (1987) for a discussion of the uses and limitations of the BDI.

Apart from the BDI, there are other measures of depression that deserve mention, such as the 20-item Zung self-rating depression scale (SDS; Zung, 1965) which has good age and sex norms (Knight, Waal-Manning & Spears, 1983) and is often easier to administer to people with limited reading ability. The major clinician-rating measure of depression is the Hamilton rating scale for depression (HRSD; Hamilton, 1960). This 17-item scale provides a means of assessing depression through an interview procedure. Many researchers have employed the interview procedure associated with the 'schedule for affective disorders and schizophrenia' (SADS; Endicott *et al.*, 1981; Endicott & Spitzer, 1978) as a means of conducting Hamilton ratings. It should be noted that the scale is heavily weighted towards the presence of physical symptoms and anxiety features, with less emphasis on the cognitive and behavioural aspects of depression. The HRSD is especially useful in situations in which a self-report scale cannot be administered (e.g. due to language difficulties or extreme psychomotor retardation) or where the self-report may be susceptible to the demands of the assessment context or other influences. Validity data for the HRSD are further discussed in a paper by Knesevich, Biggs, Clayton & Ziegler (1977).

There are numerous other devices for the assessment of depression that have much to recommend them, such as the 'Carroll rating scale' (Carroll, Feinberg, Smouse, Rawson & Greden, 1981), the 'center for epidemiological studies depression scale' (Radloff, 1977) and the recently developed 'inventory for depressive symptomatology' (Rush, Giles, Schlesser, Fulton, Weissenberger & Burns, 1986). Zimmerman and Coryell (1987) have also produced a 22-item self-report scale to be used to diagnose major depressive disorder according to DSM-III criteria. A brief review of the various depression assessment devices is available in Rehm (1981). Rather more detailed discussion of the psychometric properties of the tests can be found in Boyle (1985). A more complete overview is provided in the book by Sartorius & Ban (1986).

Assessment of mood

There are also various self-report methods for the assessment of *mood*, as distinct from the broad depressive symptomatology. One of the most widely employed is the 'depression affect adjective checklists' (DACL; Lubin, 1965), which, with its seven parallel forms, is ideal for situations requiring repeated measurement, and can therefore be used to monitor progress during the course of treatment. Another useful mood-monitoring measure involves having clients record their mood at the end of each day on a simple 10-point scale (cf Wilson, Goldin & Charbonneau-Powis, 1983 and Baker & Wilson, 1985) such as the one contained in Table 3.1.

Table 3.1: *Mood recording form*

DAY .... DATE ....

Today, on average my mood was:

Circle one:	1	2	3	4	5	6	7	8	9
	Low				Medium				Really great

Today, my worst mood was: Time: ....

What were you doing? ....

What were you thinking about? ....

....

Circle one to indicate your mood at the time:

1	2	3	4	5	6	7	8	9
Low				Medium				Really great

Today, my best mood was: Time: ....

What were you doing? ....

What were you thinking about? ....

....

Circle one to indicate your mood at the time:

1	2	3	4	5	6	7	8	9
Low				Medium				Really great

The ratings of the best, worst and average mood for each day have the advantage of yielding valuable information about the variation in mood and the conjunction with events and cognitions. A review of the psychometric properties of the various mood measures is provided by Howarth & Schokman-Gates (1981).

Measures of cognition

Beck's cognitive theory of depression has resulted in the development of a number of measures designed to provide assessments of the concepts related to his theory. Some of these measures may be useful in providing information about the nature of the person's negative thoughts. These measures include the 'dysfunctional attitude scale' (DAS; Weissman & Beck, 1978), the 'automatic thoughts questionnaire' (ATQ; Hollon & Kendall, 1980), and the 'attributional style questionnaire' (ASQ; Seligman, Abramson, Semmel & von Bayer, 1979). The DAS consists of several versions: a 100-item, and two 40-item parallel forms. Psychometric properties are presented in papers by Dobson & Breiter (1983) and Oliver & Baumgart (1985). The ATQ consists of 30 items designed to assess the frequency with which negative thoughts have been experienced during the previous week. The ASQ was designed to provide an assessment of the extent to which individuals make attributions about good and bad events in accordance with the revised learned helplessness hypothesis of depression. For each of the 12 events listed on the questionnaire (six positive, six negative), respondents are required to indicate the likely cause of the event and to provide ratings that correspond with attributions along the internal – external, global – specific and stable – unstable dimensions. Other cognitive assessment devices include the 'cognitive bias questionnaire' (CBQ; Krantz & Hammen, 1979), the 'cognitions questionnaire' (Fennell & Campbell, 1984) and the 'cognitive style questionnaire' (CSQ; Wilkinson & Blackburn, 1981). The latter scale consists of 30 items, each of which involves the description of a hypothetical situation with a choice of four possible cognitive responses from which the person has to choose the one that he/she would be most likely to think if the situation actually occurred.

Other assessment devices

Several other assessment devices may be useful in the assessment of depression. The 'pleasant events schedule' (PES; MacPhillamy & Lewinsohn, 1982) is a 320-item measure of engagement in pleasant activities. This instrument can be helpful in the assessment of activity level and in the selection of activities that the client might be able to increase in frequency. Similarly, the 'unpleasant events schedule' (Lewinsohn, Mermelstein, Alexander & MacPhillamy, 1985) or the 'Hassles Scale' (Kanner, Coyne, Schaefer & Lazarus, 1981) may also be a useful as a measure of the occurrence of negative events, some of which may be contributing to the person's depression. Kavanagh & Wilson (1987) have recently developed scales that are designed to assess self-efficacy regarding control over negative thoughts, engagement in pleasant activities and the likelihood of being able to prevent a depressive reaction in relation to a set of 30 life events. The first of these scales appears to be particularly promising as predictors of treatment response.

Treatment of depression

At our present stage of knowledge, it seems appropriate to recommend that the initial assessment of depression remains fairly broadly based in order to identify the likely causal processes involved for any given individual. Selection of treatment would depend upon the outcome of this thorough assessment. Clearly, those individuals whose problem is characterised by a high level of negative cognitive distortions would be expected to constitute the most suitable candidates for cognitive therapy. On the other hand, individuals who report significant interpersonal problems that are judged by the clinician to be causally connected with depression ought to be provided with such therapies as social-skills training, social-anxiety reduction techniques or marital therapy as indicated. Of course, many clients will require a combination of appropriate approaches. A major challenge for research on depression in the coming years will be to examine the utility of the conception of treatment selection suggested here, although some work, which is supportive of this matching of individual deficits to treatment components, has been provided by McKnight, Nelson, Hayes & Jarrett (1984).

It is important to consider the possibility of referral to a medical practitioner for an assessment of the appropriateness of antidepressant medication or hospitalisation in the treatment of depression. Such a referral may be especially important when many of the so-called endogenous features are present, when the depression is particularly severe or when there are manic symptoms, delusions or other psychotic features.

The major contemporary psychological approach to the treatment of depression is cognitive-behaviour therapy. Treatment-outcome studies have supported the efficacy of such treatment in comparison to waiting list controls (Wilson *et al.*, 1983; Larcombe & Wilson, 1984), and alternative psychological treatments such as relaxation training (McLean & Hakstian, 1979) or non-directive therapy (Shaw, 1977). Cognitive therapy has been found to be at least as beneficial as antidepressant medication (Murphy, Simons, Wetzel & Lustman, 1984). Social-skills training has also been found to produce clinically significant results (Hersen, Bellack, Himmelhoch & Thase, 1984). Another approach that bears some similarity to cognitive therapy is self-control therapy (Rehm, 1977), which has been demonstrated to be effective in the treatment of depression (Fuchs & Rehm, 1977; Roth, Bielski, Jones, Parker & Osborn, 1982).

Descriptions of the therapeutic approaches to depression can be obtained from a number of sources. The book by Beck *et al.*, 1979 (*Cognitive therapy of depression*) remains the standard reference for details of the cognitive approach. Lewinsohn's psychoeducational approach, designed for group-administration is described in the book by Lewinsohn, Antonuccio, Steinmetz & Teri (1984). There is also an excellent book on more general psychological treatments by J. M. G. Williams (1984). Reviews of the treatment-outcome literature can be obtained by consulting Becker & Heimberg (1985) or the books by Rehm (1981) or Rush (1982).

4
Assessment of Obesity

General background

At first glance, the assessment of obesity may appear quite straightforward, but closer inspection reveals many problematic issues that must be considered. For example, there is much debate about the definition of obesity and this makes measurement and estimation of incidence a difficult task. Furthermore, the aetiological factors involved are extremely complex and the assessor will need to have a good understanding of the numerous physiological, environmental and behavioural determinants of obesity. This chapter explores these issues and attempts to outline a behavioural-assessment approach, which is based upon a critical evaluation of the research literature available to date.

Incidence, definition and measurement issues

It is generally accepted that obesity refers to an excess of stored body fat (Smith & Fremouw, 1987) but the majority of criteria used to classify a person as obese or non-obese are based on measures that focus on body weight rather than body fat. This tendency to equate weight with fatness has been repeatedly criticised (Bray, 1976; Powers, 1980). A person who exceeds some criteria involving weight measurement is not necessarily excessively fat. Body fat is known to be less dense than lean body tissue and in some instances, a person with high muscle weight could be classed as obese if weight-related criteria were used, despite a low proportion of body fat. Indeed, studies such as Rogers, Mahoney

& Mahoney (1980) have demonstrated body weight to be a poor predictor of body fat. Since the only direct measure of fat is from postmortem examination, the assessor is left with the choice of either using weight-related indices or indirect measures of fatness, such as skinfold thickness. Despite the problems inherent in weight-based measures of obesity, these remain the most practical for many clinicians and consideration is therefore given to their use in this chapter.

There are various measurement methods and criteria for classification of obesity that are based on weight. The most simple method is relative weight in which the degree of obesity may be determined in terms of abnormality in comparison with the normative weight for persons of the same sex, height and build within that population. This approach suffers from the problem that normative weights for a given population tend to change over time and it seems questionable to suggest that a person should be classed as obese at one point in time and not at others. For example, in the United States, the average male weight increased by 17 lbs over the period 1950 to 1975 while average height increased by 2.46 inches. Females showed minimal change in average weight during this period, while stature increased by an average of 1.9 inches (Christakis, 1975). Generally, males of a given age and height became heavier over this period, whereas females of a given height and age became lighter. Such changes within society over time make the classification of obesity using relative-weight methods of this type rather questionable.

The most widely accepted weight-based criterion for establishing the incidence of obesity involves the concept of ideal weight. The ideal weight for an individual in a given population is determined by the weight associated with the lowest mortality rates for age, height and sex. Mortality or survival rates are typically based on life-insurance data. In the US for example, the 1979 Body Build Study produced by the Society of Actuaries and Association of Life Insurance Medical Directors of America is frequently used to establish the weight associated with greatest survival rates for age, height, sex and body build. The incidence of obesity in the population is then established in relation to some arbitrarily determined percentage of weight in excess of the ideal level. For the present purposes it is suggested that a criterion of 20 per cent in excess of ideal weight is taken as the level at which a person is classified as obese. This criterion can be justified, given evidence that suggests that above this level mortality rates can be seen to gradually increase in association with increased overweight status (Sorlie, Gordon & Kannel, 1980). Mortality rates increase dramatically amongst persons who are severely overweight (Keys, 1975; Lew & Garfinkel, 1979) but there is little evidence of increased mortality amongst individuals who are less than 20 per cent over ideal weight. Most research studies have taken 20 per cent over ideal weight as the criterion for obesity and if this definition is accepted, between 9 per cent and 37 per cent of males and 21 to 49 per cent of females in Western cultures can be regarded as weighing more than they should weigh (see Ley, 1980 for a review).

If ideal weight measurements are to be used, the assessor will need to obtain actuarial-type tables for mortality rates, which are generally available from government health departments and/or large life insurance companies. Ideal weight should take into account the person's sex, height and body build. Percentage overweight is then determined by the equation:

$$\text{Percentage overweight} = \frac{[\text{actual weight} - \text{ideal weight}] \times 100}{\text{ideal weight}}$$

One difficulty with this method is the lack of reliable means of establishing a person's body-build category. Beumont, Al-Alami & Touyz (1987) criticise the use of actuarial tables in which the method of assessing body frame is unclear and suggest the use of 'Quetelet's body mass index', which is not dependent upon body-frame measurement. The body mass index (BMI) is calculated by the equation:

$$\text{Body mass index} = \frac{\text{weight (in kilograms)}}{\text{height}^2 \text{ (in metres)}}$$

This equation is based on the premiss that tall people are generally heavier than short people and as such, represents a rather crude measure of obesity. Individuals are then categorised as obese if they exceed some criteria for BMI. This may be set in terms of deviation from the norm or to correspond with degree of overweight in comparison with ideal weight from actuarial tables. Various cut-off points for BMI are therefore used. The National Heart Foundation of Australia for example, uses a cut off of BMI>30 to label both males and females as obese. If BMI's are calculated, however, to correspond with levels such as 20 per cent above ideal weight for a given sex, height, age and body build, some of the inadequacies of BMI are revealed. For example, the BMI corresponding with 20 per cent above ideal weight for female 1.47m (4ft 10in) tall ranges from 25.5 for a small-framed woman to 33 for a large-framed woman (see Table 4.1). Hence, there is a danger of misclassifying individuals if the BMI>30 criterion is used. (These calculations are based on figures presented by the 1979 Body Build Study referred to previously.) It seems that, if body mass index is to be used as a criteria for obesity, body frame should be taken into account. The problem still remains, however, as to methods of accurately assessing a person's body build. Assuming this can be achieved, it is possible to use Table 4.1 to determine the BMI that corresponds with 20 per cent above ideal weight for a given sex, height and body build. It would be preferable also to take into account the person's age, as mean weights for height typically decline with age. Unfortunately, this information is not generally presented in actuarial tables.

Various other weight-based measurement methods are available and are summarised by Powers (1980) and Grande (1975) who discuss alternative means of assessing body fat, such as water-displacement techniques. In this chapter we focus only on those methods that are most likely to be available to the practitioner. Skinfold measures represent an indirect index of fatness that is frequently used in the research literature and may be a feasible means of assessment for some therapists. Skinfold thickness, as a measure of obesity, is based on the premiss that around 50 per cent of body fat is stored subcutaneously. Various norms for skinfold measures exist (Frisancho, 1981; Seltzer & Mayer, 1965) and again the criteria for obese status are arbitrarily set, for example, using an index of 1 standard deviation from the mean for age or sex. Various sites can be used for measurement but Franzini & Grimes (1976) suggest the use of four skinfold sites to reduce the possibility of errors in classification if only one site is taken. These authors recommend the use of subscapular, biceps, suprailiac and triceps sites. Adequate training in the use of skinfold calipers is essential, and even this does not necessarily overcome the problem of poor reliability of measurement (Durnin, Armstrong & Womersley, 1973). The assessor should therefore be cautious in the use of skinfold measures. Although many authors point out that skinfold thickness correlates better with other indices of fatness than do measures that are based on weight (Grande, 1975), it may be better to stick to more reliable methods such as percentage

Table 4.1: *Body mass index (BMI) corresponding to 120 per cent of ideal weight according to height, frame and sex*

Females				Males			
Height	BMI corresponding to 120% of ideal weight level			Height	BMI corresponding to 120% of ideal weight level		
(metres)	Small frame	Med. frame	Large frame	(metres)	Small frame	Med. frame	Large frame
1.47	25.58–27.84	27.34–30.35	29.59–32.85	1.57	28.09–29.41	28.75–30.95	30.29–32.92
1.50	24.96–27.39	26.90–29.81	29.08–32.48	1.60	27.63–28.91	28.27–30.40	29.76–32.52
1.52	24.37–26.95	26.48–29.53	28.59–32.11	1.63	27.19–28.42	27.81–29.87	29.25–32.13
1.55	24.03–27.75	26.07–29.25	28.34–31.74	1.65	26.76–27.96	27.36–29.55	28.76–31.95
1.57	23.70–26.56	25.90–28.97	28.09–31.39	1.68	26.34–27.50	26.92–29.25	28.28–31.76
1.60	23.60–26.36	25.72–28.70	27.85–31.25	1.70	25.94–27.25	26.69–28.94	28.00–31.57
1.63	23.48–26.16	25.54–28.42	27.60–31.10	1.73	25.54–27.00	26.46–28.65	27.73–31.38
1.65	23.36–25.96	25.36–28.16	27.36–30.95	1.75	25.16–26.76	26.23–28.35	27.47–31.01
1.68	23.24–25.76	25.18–27.89	27.12–30.80	1.78	24.79–26.52	26.00–28.07	27.20–30.99
1.70	23.12–25.56	25.00–27.63	26.88–30.63	1.80	24.44–26.28	25.77–27.78	26.95–30.80
1.73	22.99–25.36	24.81–27.37	26.64–30.47	1.83	24.25–26.04	25.55–27.67	26.69–30.60
1.75	22.86–25.16	24.63–27.11	26.40–30.13	1.85	24.06–25.96	25.33–27.55	26.60–30.40
1.78	22.73–24.97	24.45–26.86	26.17–29.79	1.88	23.88–25.88	25.27–27.42	26.50–30.35
1.80	22.59–24.77	24.27–26.61	25.94–29.46	1.91	23.70–25.80	25.05–27.30	26.40–30.30
1.83	22.46–24.57	24.09–26.37	25.71–29.13	1.93	23.66–25.71	24.98–27.31	26.44–30.24

Note: These figures are adapted from the 1979 Build Study of Actuaries and Association of Life Insurance Medical Directors of America, 1980.

overweight unless you are confident as to your skills in skinfold measurement. If adequate training in caliper usage is available, further guidelines can be found in Powers (1980, Ch. 1). Skinfold measures, while having the advantage of being more closely related to degree of fatness than weight-based measures, still do not overcome the problem of how to define obese status. The problem still remains as to what degree of fatness should be labelled obese and again the potential variation in the criterion for obesity makes estimation of the incidence of obesity a difficult task.

Perhaps the best method of estimating the incidence of obese status, despite the considerable limitations involved, is the use of the cut off of 20 per cent above ideal weight for age, height and body build, based on lowest mortality rates. At least this method has some socially valid reason for selecting cut-off points. Even so, studies have produced widely varying estimates of the incidence of obese status, depending on the characteristics of the sample concerned. When a client presents in the clinic, the question of whether or not he or she is obese can now be seen to be a difficult one. The client's age, sex, body build, height and culture must all be borne in mind. The issue as to whether the client would benefit from a fat-reducing programme then becomes the next tricky question. Here, a variety of other factors must be considered, such as self-perceptions of fatness, cultural and social pressures that may all influence the client's decision to seek help. These points will be dealt with in subsequent sections.

Adverse consequences of obesity

Various adverse physical and psychological consequences are suggested to be associated with obese status (Ley, 1980) and these may trigger clients to request weight-control programmes. (Note: although it is acknowledged here that weight cannot be equated with fatness, the terms weight reduction and weight control will be used to reflect attempts to reduce obese status.) For many obese people, the fear of long-term health consequences is a powerful motivating factor in the decision to seek help. Numerous health problems, such as hypertension, hyperlipidemia, diabetes mellitus, pulmonary and renal problems, have been suggested to be associated with obese status (Van Itallie, 1979). As mentioned previously, the incidence of adverse health effects seems to increase as percentage over ideal weight increases, once a level of

20 per cent excess is surpassed. Interestingly, minimal attention seems to have been paid to the potential health hazards of underweight individuals, with researchers and practitioners tending to focus on overweight issues unless the degree of underweight is sufficiently severe to warrant classification of anorexia nervosa. It must be acknowledged that the nature of the association between obese status and adverse health effects is unclear. Some authors such as Smith & Fremouw (1987) point out that the effect of obesity on health may result from the adverse psychological influence of society upon obese individuals rather than there being a direct physical relationship. These authors cite a study by Stout, Morrow, Brandt & Wolf (1964), which was conducted with an Italian–American community where obesity was regarded as socially acceptable. The incidence of heart disease and diabetes mellitus was actually below the US national average despite a high level of obesity. This evidence does raise the issue of whether treatment efforts should be geared towards weight reduction or to the shifting of negative societal attitudes towards obesity, combined with encouraging obese persons to cope more effectively with any persecution they receive. Until the nature of the relationship between obesity and health is clarified, however, it would seem sensible to assume a direct relationship and continue attempts at weight reduction for individuals whose weight exceeds 20 per cent of ideal levels. Little case exists on health grounds for intervention with clients who exceed ideal weight up to this 20 per cent level. In our physique-conscious society, the motivation to cut down on fat storage is often cosmetic, particularly amongst women (Ley, 1980). The therapist may therefore be faced with a dilemma as to whether to facilitate weight-reduction attempts with marginally overweight individuals.

Studies have also suggested that obese persons are more likely than non-obese people to experience a range of adverse psychosocial difficulties (Allon, 1982; Brownell, 1982; Ley, 1980). Smith & Fremouw (1987) suggest that these result from society's pervasive negative attitude towards obesity. It should be pointed out, however, that there are marked cultural differences in attitude towards weight status and most studies have focused on white, Anglo-Saxon populations. Undoubtedly, individuals differ in the degree to which they experience psychosocial problems as the result of being overweight. Reviews of the literature (see Ley, 1980; Brownell, 1982) typically conclude that, generally, obese persons are more likely to be perceived as possessing negative attributes than their non-obese counterparts, and to receive unfavourable outcomes from situations such as interviews. Certainly, many obese clients report that a major reason for seeking help is to enable them to feel more attractive to others. Where clients report such feelings, it seems appropriate to take such issues seriously.

Aetiological factors in obesity

A wide variety of biological, psychological and environmental factors appear to be involved in the development and maintenance of obesity (LeBow, 1984). Whatever the reason for obese status, it is generally accepted that fat storage results from an imbalance between energy intake and expenditure. When caloric intake exceeds expenditure, the remaining energy is converted to fat and stored within adipose tissue (LeBow, 1984). Various reasons for this state of affairs have been proposed.

Genetic factors

Genetic factors have been suggested to be involved for some individuals in the determination of metabolic rate and number of adipocytes (Foch & McClearn, 1980), which in turn influence the level of fat deposits. A recent study of adopted children conducted by Stunkard, Sorenson, Hanis, Teasdale, Chakrabarty, Schull & Schulsinger (1986) supported the role of hereditary influences in obesity. A clear relation between weight class of adoptees and the Body Mass Index of their biological parents was found, but no relation was evident with the BMI of adoptive parents. Genetic influences therefore emerged as being stronger than environmental factors in the determination of weight status. The presence of genetic influences in obesity does not necessarily indicate physiological rather than behavioural determinants. It is also feasible that hereditary influences may be present in relation to activity levels and eating habits. Much more research is needed to clarify the role of hereditary factors and meanwhile the search for behavioural and environmental influences should continue.

Set-point theory

Even if genetic factors are involved in the development and

maintenance of obesity it is important to explore how these factors operate. Set-point theory represents one attempt to explain why many individuals find it so difficult to lose weight despite rigorous attempts at dieting. Keesey (1980) points out that individuals are remarkably consistent in weight over time and that weight-reduction attempts are frequently unsuccessful in the long term. He proposes that each person has some biologically programmed ideal weight (set point) and a series of regulatory processes act to maintain this body weight by adjusting energy intake and expenditure (by adjusting exercise levels and metabolic rate). Hence, if a person cuts down his caloric intake by dieting, there is a tendency for activity levels and metabolic rate to compensate by slowing down to keep body weight constant. From a survival perspective, this process makes sense in that the system would facilitate survival at times of reduced food availability. There is considerable evidence to suggest that, as caloric intake decreases, metabolic rate tends to decline (Keesey, 1980) and an increase in the efficiency of food utilisation occurs, which encourages the storage of fat (Smith & Fremouw, 1987). Little is known about ways of preventing this homeostatic process from operating, but the model does explain why so many people find that dieting produces so little weight reduction.

Dieting as a perpetuator of obesity

Recent authors have suggested that not only is dieting often minimally effective in producing fat loss, but it may also serve to maintain obesity in some individuals. For example, Smith & Fremouw (1987) present evidence to suggest that severe dietary restriction may act to reduce lean tissue as well as fat deposits, which in turn leads to a further reduction in metabolic rate as fat tissue tends to burn up less energy than lean tissue. Furthermore, Garrow (1974) reported that the reduction in energy expenditure that tends to accompany dieting becomes more efficient with repeated dieting attempts. Repeated dieters therefore require fewer and fewer calories to lose the same amount of weight with each attempt and this may explain why a history of dieting is associated with poor prognosis (Smith & Fremouw, 1987). One method of counteracting the metabolic slowdown is to encourage a heavy-exercise programme (Brownell, 1982), which is suggested to increase the proportion of higher energy-burning lean tissue and to reduce appetite.

Certain types of diets have also been suggested to result in binge eating and adverse psychological reactions. High-fat, low-bulk diets, for example, have been linked with carbohydrate cravings and binge eating (Smith & Fremouw, 1987) and these authors propose the use of low-fat, high-bulk diets to counteract this possibility. Furthermore, some researchers (e.g. Stunkard, 1983; Halmi, Stunkard & Mason, 1980) report increases in depression and anxiety symptoms as the results of dieting attempts. Contradictory findings, however, are reported by Ley (1984) but differences in the dietary regimes used in these studies may possibly account for the different results. The possible link between dieting and adverse emotional reactions has led to the proposition that dieting may trigger further episodes of overeating as a means of reducing negative affect in individuals who are prone to overeat at such times (Smith & Fremouw, 1987). Evidence does suggest that many people tend to overeat when they are feeling distressed (Lowe & Fisher, 1983). Such hypotheses should certainly be borne in mind during assessment as such cycles of dieting, negative affect, overeating and dieting may be evident for some individuals.

Hyperplastic versus hypertrophic status

The composition of a person's fat deposits may also influence the development and maintenance of obesity. The amount of fat stored in the body is determined by both the number and the size of fat cells (adipocytes). It was traditionally held that increases in numbers of fat cells occurred mainly during childhood and once puberty was reached, increased fat storage resulted mainly from an increase in the size of existing cells. This position is now thought to be an oversimplification, with evidence that fat cells may also multiply in adulthood once a certain increase in existing fat cell size has been achieved (Bjorntorp & Sjostrom, 1971). It was also previously held that individuals with a higher-than-average number of fat cells (i.e. hyperplastic, and by implication, child-onset obesity) find it harder to reduce fat storage down to normal levels than those with a normal number of fat cells that are enlarged in size (i.e. hypertropic, and by implication, adult-onset obesity). Here again, evidence is conflicting. Bjornorp, Carlgren, Isaksson, Krotkiewski, Larsson & Sjornstrom (1975) reported that, as women lost weight, their progress ceased once their fat cells reach normal size. Hence, women with an increased number of fat cells were suggested to be at a disadvantage and indeed tended to remain overweight after treatment. It was suggested that, although their fat cells reduced to normal size, the larger number of fat cells meant that they were still overweight after treatment in many cases. For women with a normal number of fat cells, the reduction in cell size to normal levels during treatment allowed them to attain normal weight levels.

Indirect evidence in support of the hyperplastic/hypertroptic model was also presented by Colvin & Olson (1983) who suggested that adult-onset obesity has a better prognosis than child- or adolescent-onset obesity. A recent study reported by Strain, Strain, Zurnoff & Knittle (1984), however, brings the hyperplastic/hypertrophic model into question. These authors found that many individuals were both hyperplastic and hypertrophic and that fat-cell morphometrics did not predict successful weight reduction. The evidence is therefore conflicting and the model awaits further clarification.

Maladaptive eating and exercise habits

The majority of behaviour-therapy approaches to weight reduction are based on a series of questionable assumptions regarding the maladaptive eating and exercise habits of obese persons. First, it has been assumed that obese individuals eat excessively, particularly in relation to high-calorie foods. The second assumption is that overweight people tend to eat more in response to external stimuli rather than to internal hunger cues compared to their non-obese counterparts. Third, it has also been assumed that overweight persons engage in excessively low levels of activity. Intervention has therefore aimed to reduce caloric intake by means of dietary education, self-monitoring, the setting of lowered calorie-intake goals, the breaking of stimulus-control patterns so as to bring eating under 'self control' and finally, increasing exercise levels through aerobic activity and changes in life style. For some individuals, this approach is successful but the long-term results of many behavioural programmes have not been encouraging (Foreyt & Kondo, 1984). Weight losses in behavioural programmes rarely exceed 8 kg, which represents only a fraction of the excess weight of most persons seeking treatment (Wadden & Stunkard, 1986). The minimal weight reduction achieved may be due to the invalidity of the assumptions upon which traditional behaviour-therapy approaches are based, at least as far as many clients are concerned. For example, there is little evidence from observational studies to support the view that overweight persons consume more calories than non-obese persons (Wooley, Wooley & Dyrenforth, 1979) but it is feasible that obese persons tend to eat more when they are alone or in other situations where observations are not typically made. Perhaps they also tend to finish food selected or seek out food locations where more calories are served. Indeed Stunkard & Mazer (1978) report that obese people are overrepresented at smorgasbords, which supports this latter suggestion. Although research to date has not supported differences between obese and non-obese people in food intake or even in eating style, it seems likely that the relevant behavioural dimensions have not yet been explored, given evidence from metabolic studies that obese persons ingest more calories than their non-obese counterparts (Bray, 1976).

The evidence supporting the notion that obesity is associated with external stimulus control of eating is also variable. This model was proposed by Stunkard & Koch (1964) and suggests that obese persons tend to eat in response to external stimuli, such as sight of food, rather than in response to the internal stimuli of hunger. In support of this theory, Brownell (1981) outlines evidence to suggest that obese persons are more responsive to time they think has passed rather than actual time, to visual properties of food and to palatability of food than non-obese people. There is little evidence, however, to suggest that obese persons eat more frequently during other activities, e.g. watching TV or reading than do normal weight people, and these activities are the typical targets of many behavioural programmes that use stimulus-control methods. Similarly, with regard to eating style, research to date has failed to demonstrate that overweight people eat faster or chew less compared to non-obese persons, although these areas are often targeted during behavioural assessment and treatment.

Given the variable evidence for stimulus-control determinants of obesity, it is strange that so many behavioural programmes incorporate stimulus-control modification components into treatment and even more surprising that in some instances, they produce weight loss even when used in isolation from other methods (Weiss, 1977). Perhaps the reason that stimulus-control procedures and modification of eating style have been successful in producing weight loss is that they encourage an overall reduction in food intake by limiting the places in, and the rate at which, food can be eaten. It is worth noting here that those factors that are effective in producing weight loss are not necessarily implicated in the determination or maintenance of excess fat storage. When stimulus-control approaches are effective in producing weight reduction, this may be through mechanisms other than the change in maladaptive external control patterns. Effectiveness does not necessarily imply that obese people differ from non-obese individuals in terms of stimulus control in the first place.

A similar picture of confusion emerges when activity levels are considered. Although many studies have shown that obese persons typically engage in lower activity levels (Stern, 1984), other studies have indicated that because they weigh more, obese people actually burn up just as many calories as the non-obese, given that they have to expend more energy per given activity (Lutwak & Coulston, 1975). Brownell (1981) suggests that it is likely that, overall, obese persons use up marginally less energy than non-obese people, despite the need for higher burn-up rates for a given activity, thereby tipping the balance in favour of fat storage. Until evidence is produced from prolonged naturalistic studies, firm conclusions cannot be drawn.

As mentioned previously, it is also likely that exercise has an important role to play in the maintenance of obesity through the influence on proportion of lean body tissue. If, as Smith and Fremouw (1987) suggest, fat tissue tends to use up less energy than lean tissue, the greater proportion of fat: lean tissue that exists for obese persons would tend to make it more likely that excess energy will remain and be stored as fat. To reduce this problem, a relatively greater proportion of lean tissue compared to fat needs to be created in order to increase energy usage both during resting metabolism and exercise. Exercise tends to increase the ratio of lean tissue to fat and is therefore suggested to be an important component of fat-reduction programmes. Furthermore, Brownell (1981) suggests that, contrary to general belief, exercise tends to reduce appetite rather than enhance it, which provides additional support for exercise as a component of weight-reduction regimes. Research studies do support the value of exercise, particularly in enhancing the long-term benefits of behavioural weight-control programmes (Harris & Hallbauer, 1973; Stalonas, Johnson & Christ, 1978).

Summary regarding aetiological factors

The discussion of aetiological determinants of obesity albeit brief, presents a complicated picture in which each client brings to treatment a different set of genetic, biological, environmental and behavioural influences. Identification of those variables that are relevant to designing an individually tailored treatment programme is important. Such information may also allow prediction of response to treatment and selection of an approach most likely to be effective. It should be borne in mind that different factors may operate in the initial development as compared to current maintenance of obese status. Although evidence is conflicting, and in some cases far from convincing, it does seem that a multiplicity of factors are involved in the development and maintenance of obesity. In particular, assessment should consider the role of physiological determinants, dietary intake, eating habits, exercise levels, influences of negative affect and the possible perpetuating effects of repeated dieting. The behavioural interview presented in this chapter aims to take this type of multifaceted perspective in order to identify the relevant factors for each client. It may be helpful first to consider the use of other psychological assessment measures that may be useful in the process.

Specific assessment measures

Various methods of self-monitoring and questionnaires for completion by the client or relevant others may be used to supplement the information produced by the behavioural interview. In particular, self-monitoring is a useful means of exploring the client's eating and exercise habits and of identifying relevant antecedent conditions and consequences of overeating. For example, specific situations that trigger negative affect and/or overeating may be pinpointed for some clients, as may negative emotional response to overeating. Clients may also be asked to monitor caloric intake, in which case small calorie-counting books are available quite cheaply from many book shops. Clients will obviously vary in their accuracy of self-monitoring and some will be reluctant to look up and record actual caloric values. In such instances, it may be necessary to limit recording to food type and portion size, with caloric intake being determined by the assessor. Brownell (1984) emphasises the low accuracy of self-recording of food intake, whether on a continuous monitoring or 24-hour recall basis. It may be feasible to improve accuracy of self-monitoring by giving the client clear instructions, practice sessions in the clinic with feedback and devising a system of prompts for monitoring and recording, such as a one-hour beeper (Nay, 1979). In order to identify relevant antecedents and consequences of overeating, it is also useful to ask clients to monitor information concerning when and where they eat, how they feel before and after and other resulting events. Table 4.2 provides an example of the type of self-monitoring form that may be used.

Having obtained the information about food intake, the assessor must then decide whether it is excessive and whether reduction is required. Most national departments of health will provide tables of dietary requirements for individuals of different ages, heights and weight. Although guidelines as to appropriate diet and caloric intake are available in excellent texts such as Stuart & Davis (1972), it is recommended that dietary programmes are designed by trained dieticians, unless the assessor has a competent training in nutrition to enable design of a healthy eating programme. In addition to assessing caloric intake, it is also important to consider the balance of nutrition across the major food groups. It is feasible to avoid detailed calorie counting by the assessment of food exchanges across the major food groups (Stuart & Davis, 1972). It is important to note that self-monitoring of food intake frequently has a reactive effect, resulting in a decline in food intake (Nay, 1979). Remember then that the information may not be truly indicative of eating behaviour prior to monitoring.

The assessment of energy expenditure is also useful as few practitioners have access to accurate measurement devices to evaluate activity levels or energy consumption. Table 4.3 outlines an activity diary that can be used to record type of activity and the level of energy expenditure involved. Table 4.4 lists some common activities that may be used as a guide to determining the level of energy used in various forms of recreation and lifestyle exercise.

In addition to self-monitoring of eating and exercise levels, specific self-report instruments may be used. For example, the 'Stanford eating disorders questionnaire' (Agras *et al.*, 1976) considers the person's demographic details, weight and medical history, psychological and social functioning. Unfortunately, it is rather time-consuming to complete and data concerning its reliability is lacking. Further information concerning eating style and food preferences may also be obtained by direct observation.

Table 4.2: *Daily eating diary*

Name: Date:

Time	Where are you?	Who with?	What else are you doing?	How were you feeling before eating?	What do you eat?	How much?	How do you feel after eating?	Calorie value?

Table 4.3: *Daily exercise diary*

Name:

Date:

	Activity level in terms of energy usage (see Table 4.4)		
	Low	Medium	High
a.m. 12–1.00			
1–2.00			
2–3.00			
3–4.00			
4–5.00			
5–6.00			
6–7.00			
7–8.00			
8–9.00			
9–10.00			
10–11.00			
11–12.00			
12–1.00			
p.m. 1–2.00			
2–3.00			
3–4.00			
4–5.00			
5–6.00			
6–7.00			
7–8.00			
8–9.00			
9–10.00			
10–11.00			
11–12.00			

Note: Please record actual activity involved and time in minutes.

Table 4.4: *Level of energy expenditure for various recreation and lifestyle activities*

	Recreation	Lifestyle
High	Skiing	Walking upstairs
	Jogging	
	Canoeing	
	Sprinting	
(Greater than	Squash	
7 cals/min)	Sprinting	Skipping rope
	Rapid cycling	
	Aerobic dancing	
	Football	
	Basketball	Walking downstairs
Medium	Badminton	Fast walking
	Cycling	
4–7 cals	Dancing	Digging
per minute	Tennis	Chopping wood
	Swimming	Heavy gardening
	Waterskiing	
Low	Golf	Dressing
(less than	Baseball (except pitcher)	Sleeping
4 cals/Min)	Cricket (except bowler)	Sitting
	Table tennis	Standing
		Slow walking
		Most household chores

Note: Based on classification by Stuart and Davis (1972).

This has the disadvantages of being very costly on therapist time and possibly of influencing the behaviour of the client. Direct observation has therefore mostly been confined to research studies. It may be feasible, though, to request and train significant others in the client's life to observe and record eating and exercise habits as a means of validating client self-report.

As mentioned previously, some studies such as Halmi, Stunkard & Mason (1980) have reported adverse psychological effects consequent upon weight control programmes. Thus, there is a good case for initial assessment of anxiety and depression levels in order to have a baseline against which to monitor potential changes during treatment (see Chapters 2 and 3).

The behavioural interview

Prior to the behavioural assessment interview, it is important that all clients undergo a medical examination to consider physical disorders that may account for their obese status and that indicate a need for medical intervention. Additionally, the therapist must be assured that a behavioural weight-control programme is unlikely to adversely affect the client's health. A letter of clearance from a medical practitioner is therefore recommended before commencing the programme. The initial phase of the interview should then focus on the client's medical history, development of obese status and likely causal factors. The later stages progress to cover the behavioural factors that may have initially determined and/or are now maintaining obese status. Factors that are likely to influence response to treatment such as motivational level and expectancies should also be explored. Consideration should be given to the concept of dieting as a perpetuating phenomena of obesity. The following questions provide a guide to the behavioural assessment of adult obesity.

Historical background

Investigate the history of the client's weight problem:

Can you tell me how old you were when you first started to become overweight?

What weight are you currently?

Can you tell me about any illnesses that you have suffered either in childhood or in adulthood?

Are any other members of your family (parents, siblings, partner, children) overweight?

Since you first became overweight, has this remained a constant problem?

If there have been fluctuations, find out what weight the client has returned to, and when, and what was happening in their lives at the time and how the reduction was achieved.

Why do you think you first became overweight? Would you say that you tended to overeat at that time? Was your lifestyle very sedentary?

If the client was overweight as a child, questions concerning family eating and exercise habits in childhood may be relevant here.

Have you any ideas about why you continue to be overweight?

Dieting history and previous treatments

Have you tried dieting in your attempt to lose weight?

If relevant:

How successful has dieting been? What makes you give up on a diet? Do you find dieting makes you miserable . . . or anxious? How do you feel when you give up on your diet? What type of diet do you tend to use? (*e.g. high fibre, commercial diets, commercial products, low carbohydrate.*)

Do you calorie count? If so, what calorie limit do you set for yourself?

How good are you at sticking to your diet when you put yourself on one?

What other methods have you tried? What about exercise programmes? How successful have these methods been?

Eating habits

Can you describe for me what you would eat and drink in a typical day?

Make a list of anything consumed, including butter/margarine, sauces, snacks and drinks from waking to sleep onset. This should be recorded on an hourly basis. Ask the client to estimate the size of each portion so that you can later determine caloric intake. You can then compare this typical day with subsequent eating diaries.

What are your favourite foods? What foods do you eat most of?

What books or handouts have you read about nutrition and healthy eating? Are you aware of the different food groups, for example, meat, cereals, fruit, fats, vegetables, dairy products, and how much of each type should you eat?

Do you eat three meals a day? Do you tend to eat snacks in between meals? How often do you eat takeaway meals or eat out at fast-food places?

Are there any particular times when you eat more than usual? Can you tell me about these? (e.g. when alone, or feeling miserable or bored, or being away on trips, or when studying, or when out at dinners). How often does this happen?

Do you find you eat more if you are feeling miserable or worried?

Do you go out to many dinners or parties where it is too hard to avoid fattening foods?

If relevant ask:

At the times when you overeat are you aware of any particular thoughts that go through your head, or things that you say to yourself?

What triggers you to eat? Do you eat only when you feel hungry? What does it feel like when you are hungry? Do you eat while watching TV, or when reading, or when doing other activities?

Having explored a wide range of antecedents of eating, including environmental, cognitive and emotional factors, it is also important to explore the client's eating style and the consequences of overeating. Bear in mind that not all overweight persons eat excessively and the interviewer should refrain from over-questioning in this area with such clients.

Do you tend to eat quickly? How often do you have second helpings? Do you plan out your meals in advance? Do you try to make sure these are healthy and low in fattening foods? Do you tend to cook more food than is needed for one portion each? What do you do with the leftovers? Do you cook your food in ways that reduce the fat content, such as boiling or grilling rather than frying? How often do you eat fried foods?

Dealing with tempting situations

Do you find it hard to refuse the offer of fattening foods or second helpings?

What do you usually do in such situations? What thoughts go through your mind when you are about to be tempted?

Do you praise yourself when you have resisted the offer of fattening foods?

How do you feel when you have managed to say 'no'?

Emotional and cognitive aspects

Information has already been sought as to emotions and cognitions that precede overeating and the cognitive and emotional consequences related to overeating, dieting and weight gain/loss now require consideration, in addition to general attitude regarding weight status.

How do you feel about your weight problem? What are your thoughts about your own body? What would your ideal body be like?

What do you say to yourself after you have given in and eaten fattening foods?

How do you feel emotionally? What do you do next?

Sociocultural influences

When asking these questions, it is assumed that the assessor has taken a personal history, noting family and housing situation and culture.

What do your family feel about your coming along here?

Are they willing to support you? Do you think they would take part in any eating and exercise programmes with you?

What about any close friends . . . would they be willing to support you?

Are there any things in your family, work or social situation that you would like to change? What are these?

Do you feel that these affect your weight problem?

Exercise habits

Tables 4.3 and 4.4 can be used here.

Can you tell me about the kinds of exercise you take each week?

Can you take a typical day and we'll go through it hour by hour to work out how much exercise you are getting?

Is much of your time spent sitting or standing still — at home, at work, socially?

Do you try to avoid exercise if you can, such as going to local places in the car instead of walking, or taking the lift or escalator, to avoid a couple of flights of stairs?

Can you tell me about some areas in your daily living where you could get more exercise than you do at the moment?

What about any sports activities? What do you do at the moment? Are there any sports which you think you could start to do as a way of losing weight?

How would you feel about going along to join in this activity? What would your main worries be here?

Motivational aspects

Why did you decide to come to this programme now?

What are your main reasons for wanting to lose weight (e.g. cosmetic/health/self-concept/partner-pressure)?

How successful do you think you are going to be in losing weight this time?

What do you think may stop you from succeeding in this programme?

Asking clients to list likely reasons for failure may enable the therapist to take measures to reduce the likelihood of occurrence of such events.

What goals do you hope to achieve from this programme?

It is suggested that the interview ends on a motivating and encouraging note. Hopefully, the assessor will have established a trusting relationship with the client and this should allow the taking of weight and height measurements. The client should be weighed in the same state of dress on each subsequent occasion, and it is recommended that shoes be removed and only light clothing be worn. Similarly, height should be measured in stockinged feet, against a wall.

Comments regarding treatment

Numerous texts on the topic of eating and weight disorders have emerged in the past 10 years but the most useful practical guide to treatment probably remains the book by Stuart & Davis (1972) — *Slim chance in a fat world.* A useful review of the current status of behavioural treatments for obesity is given by Foreyt & Kondo (1984), which the reader should also find helpful. These authors conclude that treatment content has changed minimally over the past 15 years, tending to focus on self-monitoring, stimulus control, dietary and exercise targeting, nutrition education and contingency management. Generally speaking, the results of behavioural weight-control programmes have been modest and this has led to authors such as Smith & Fremouw (1987) to rethink the approach to treatment. These authors suggest that individuals with a long history of failed dieting, particularly those with early-onset obesity, would perhaps benefit more from long-term, gradual changes in eating, exercise and lifestyle habits, rather than severe dietary attempts. For those individuals for whom the more traditional behavioural regime is more likely to be helpful, i.e. adult onset, without a long history of repeated dieting (Smith & Fremouw, 1987), the role of the therapist is also to seek ways to maximise the effectiveness of treatment by enhancing compliance to treatment methods, reducing dropout and facilitating maintenance of weight reduction. These issues have been the major limitations in the effectiveness of behavioural wight-reduction programmes (Foreyt & Kondo, 1984). A recent shift has also been evident towards the use of very low-calorie diets. Wadden & Stunkard (1986) demonstrated that a combination of behavioural therapy and very low-calorie diet produced significantly greater weight reduction than either method alone and the result (19.3 kg loss) was considerably more than the average (8 kg) lost in behavioural programmes in general. Furthermore, reasonable maintenance of losses was evident at a one-year follow-up. Generally, the use of the very low-calorie diets is not recommended without the existence of close medical supervision, which makes the approach unsuitable for many behaviour-therapy programmes (Foreyt & Kondo, 1984).

It is interesting that the majority of behavioural weight-control programmes reported in the literature tend to use a package approach to treatment. We suggest here that the mediocre results of many behavioural treatments to date are due to the failure to tailor intervention to the characteristics of the individual. A carefully conducted assessment should enable the therapist to identify the variables that are currently maintaining the client's obese status, whether they be physiological, environmental or psychological. Intervention should then aim to influence those maintaining variables through environmental and behaviour change. What is very clear is that the behavioural assessor/therapist requires a detailed knowledge of the biological mechanisms involved in weight control and their interaction with behaviour. Furthermore, intervention requires competency in the area of nutrition and these points should be borne in mind by those considering the implementation of behavioural weight-control programmes.

5

Assessment of Interpersonal Problems

Introduction

Problems relating to interpersonal functioning are extremely common amongst clients seeking the help of mental-health professionals. Bryant, Trower, Yardley, Urbieta & Letemendia (1976) for example, report that around 16 per cent of psychiatric outpatients may be judged as experiencing interpersonal problems. The nature of the presenting problem, however, may vary considerably. In some instances, the client may seek help following adverse consequences from certain social situations, such as a failure to obtain or to remain in employment, or difficulty in forming friendships. Alternatively, or additionally, the client may be avoiding specific social situations as the result of feelings of discomfort. Social problems such as these are not necessarily the main reason a client seeks help. In many cases, problems of social functioning come to light following referral relating to some other difficulty, such as depression, agoraphobia or alcohol abuse. Indeed, evidence of difficulty in interpersonal functioning has been found in relation to a wide range of psychological disorders, including schizophrenia (Bellack & Hersen, 1978), depression (Youngren & Lewinsohn, 1980), drug abuse (Callner & Ross, 1976) and sexual deviancy (Barlow, Abel, Blanchard, Bristow & Young, 1977). Whether social problems represent a cause or effect of these conditions remains to be conclusively demonstrated. Some evidence does exist, however, to suggest that a person's level of social functioning has important implications in relation to frequency of hospitalisation, response to treatment and post-hospital adjustment for a variety of psychological disorders (Lowe, 1982;

Schooler & Spohn, 1982; Zigler & Phillips, 1961). This provides a good case for interventions designed to improve interpersonal functioning as a preventative measure and as part of the remediation process in mental-health programmes.

As with the assessment of any psychological disorder, the first step is to determine whether a problem does exist and to clarify the nature of the problem, prior to exploring the causal factors. It is important to note that the client is not always aware of the existence of social problems, which, in many cases, will emerge as being secondary to some other referral problem. Alternatively, it may be a family member, a nurse or some other professional who makes the request for intervention. For practical purposes, a social problem can be said to exist if the client experiences strong subjective discomfort in certain social situations, avoids certain interactions or fails to obtain desired and/or culturally acceptable outcomes from social encounters in a manner judged by relevant others to be acceptable. Once it has been established that some problem relating to social functioning exists, the nature and determinants of the problem must be considered.

Factors influencing social functioning

The reasons why a person may experience interpersonal problems are manifold. It may be that the person does not possess the necessary skills to perform competently. Alternatively, these skills may exist but may be inhibited for some reason. Furthermore, the explanation may relate to factors beyond the individual, such as unrealistic expectations of others or inappropriate responding by others. The following sections attempt to outline some of the major determinants of social functioning that should be considered during the assessment process.

Social skills

Ladd & Mize (1983) define social skills as the 'ability to organize cognitions and behaviours into an integrated course of action directed towards culturally acceptable social or interpersonal goals' (p. 127). This definition includes the ability to continuously assess and modify goal-directed behaviour so as to maximise the likelihood of reaching one's goals. These authors, and others such as Argyle & Kendon (1967) and McFall (1982), have outlined detailed models of the processes involved in determining exactly what a person does in a social situation. Many of these processes will be discussed here, but the extent to which formal assessment of each area is feasible is very variable, depending on the current status of research.

Argyle & Kendon (1967) stress the importance of the person's motivation and goals in determining the nature of social responding. Adequate responding also requires the individual to be able to perceive and interpret social information from the outside world correctly, in particular, the meaning of other peoples' nonverbal cues (Morrison & Bellack, 1981). A further series of cognitive processes are then involved in what Spivack & Shure (1976) term 'interpersonal problem-solving'. In order to behave appropriately in a given social interaction, individuals must be able to interpret the social context correctly, to generate ideas regarding possible alternative responses, to predict likely consequences and to select the most suitable course of action.

Assuming the client is able to complete these stages satisfactorily, it is then necessary to be able to integrate a wide range of very specific microresponses and sequence them appropriately. This is essential if the chosen response strategy is to be performed in a manner that would be judged as adequate by others. It is this aspect of social skills that has received the most attention in the research literature, with numerous studies focusing on the training of various non-verbal and paralinguistic microskills (e.g. Hersen & Bellack, 1976; Linden & Wright, 1980). This approach emphasises the need to increase appropriate usage of a wide range of microresponses, such as eye contact, tone of voice, facial expression, posture, gesture and latency of responding. By making the clients aware of the importance of such behaviours, and providing them with modelling experiences and the opportunity to practise and receive feedback, it is assumed that those skills will improve and be applied in subsequent naturalistic interactions. The improvement in appropriate microskill usage is proposed to lead to more successful outcomes from social interactions and the client being judged more favourably by others. Ultimately, it is anticipated that appropriate microskill usage will become 'automatic', being controlled by a level of cognitive processing where one is unaware of its occurrence (Argyle & Kendon, 1967). Table 5.1 outlines some of the basic and complex skill areas typically considered during social-skills training programmes.

It is beyond the scope of this chapter to outline the enormous number of cognitive and behavioural skills that have been

Table 5.1: *Examples of basic social-skill areas*

Verbal	*Non-verbal*
Tone and pitch of voice	Social distance
Volume	Posture
Fluency	Gestures
Rate of speech	Facial expression
Latency of response	Body movements
Clarity	Eye contact
Amount spoken	
Verbal listening skills	
e.g. acknowledgement	
question feedback	

Examples of complex social-skill areas

	In dealing with:
Integration of basic skills	Starting conversations
	Ending conversations
	Maintaining conversations
	Dealing with criticism
	Listening to others
	Giving praise/compliments/affection
	Giving criticisms
	Making requests
	Refusing requests

suggested to be prerequisites of appropriate social behaviour. Table 5.2 however, attempts to outline the major cognitive-skill areas that should be considered during assessment. The reader is also referred to comprehensive texts such as Hargie, Saunders & Dickson (1981) or Trower (1984). The main point that is emphasised in this chapter is the need for the assessor to consider a wide range of possible sources of breakdown in social-skill performance. In many instances, however, the client may be found to have all the necessary skills within his or her cognitive-behavioural repertoire and yet, for some reason, embarks on an inappropriate course of action or avoids specific social situations. The assessment process must then explore why this is the case.

Affect control and maladaptive cognitions

Arkowitz (1981) suggests that for some clients, appropriate cognitive-behavioural social-skill usage may be inhibited. The client may possess good social knowledge and demonstrate competent use of microskills in some circumstances, and yet behave

Table 5.2: *Cognitive processes involved in determining social responding*

(a) *Social perception* (see Morrison & Bellack, 1981)

Receiving information from others and environment relevant to the interaction

Attention to relevant aspects of information received

Knowledge of social rules

Knowledge of the significance or meaning of various responses

Correct interpretation of information received

Perspective taking ability

(b) *Social problem-solving skills* (see Spivack & Shure, 1976)

Identification of the nature and existence of a problem situation to be solved and aims of all involved

Generating ideas regarding possible alternative responses

Predicting likely consequences of each course of action (requires knowledge of social rules and behaviours required in different situations)

Selecting the response most likely to lead to desired consequence

Searching own repertoire for a similar response

Generating new repertoires of responding

Plan and sequence a wide range of responses to execute selected course of action

(c) *Self-monitoring*

Observe and correctly perceive outcome of own actions, and response of others

Adjust responses where appropriate

Accurate labelling of own behaviour

in a manner during certain social situations that is judged by others to be inappropriate. Alternatively, the client may know exactly what to do and theoretically is able to perform competently and yet avoids certain social situations as the result of feelings of discomfort. One possible explanation of social avoidance or response inhibition is that the individual experiences high levels of conditioned anxiety associated with specific social situations (Curran, 1977). As with any phobic disorder, the assessment process should consider the motoric, physiological and cognitive-response components of the anxiety and related behaviour (Bellack, 1979). Intervention should then tackle each aspect, increasing exposure to avoided situations, teaching control over physiological components through relaxation training and enhancing adaptive cognitions relating to the problem. It has been suggested by some authors that, by reducing the anxiety associated with the feared social situation, the individual will automatically increase appropriate usage of social skills, assuming these responses are within the client's repertoire but are inhibited (Trower, Yardley, Bryant & Shaw, 1978). These authors present evidence to suggest that socially anxious individuals respond favourably to both exposure and social-skills training approaches. These findings are explained by proposing that social-skills training also provides a desensitising experience for phobic individuals, who are encouraged to use their previously inhibited skills in a non-threatening situation. In reality, a combined skills-training – anxiety-reduction approach is likely to be most useful for socially anxious clients, in order to ensure the presence of an adequate social-skills repertoire and provide an exposure experience.

In addition to the emotional and behavioural aspects of social anxiety, it is important to consider the cognitions involved during social interactions. Evidence suggests that a variety of maladaptive cognitions may inhibit social performance (Alden & Saffran, 1978; Gormally, Sipps, Raphael, Edwin & Varvil-Wald, 1981). This has implications for treatment in that cognitive restructuring may be necessary to reduce maladaptive cognitions and enhance more appropriate thoughts (Stefanek & Eisler, 1983). Rathjen (1980) summarises a range of maladaptive cognitive processes that may inhibit appropriate social responding. These include irrational beliefs and distorted thinking processes such as arbitrary inference, magnification, overgeneralisation, dichotomous reasoning and catastrophising. Distorted attributions, faulty self-appraisal and irrational values and expectancies are also suggested to interfere with social performance.

Overall then, it is proposed that any model of social functioning should consider fully the possible involvement of inhibitory mechanisms. There seems little point in spending considerable time teaching sophisticated social-skills if the person is not going to use them as the result of competing anxiety or maladaptive thoughts.

Personal characteristics

The decision to label an individual's social performance as competent or incompetent is influenced by numerous factors over and above what a person actually does. Rathjen (1980) emphasises that such decisions are greatly influenced by the personal characteristics of the performer. Factors such as age, sex, culture, socioeconomic level, physical appearance, mode of dress and grooming are all suggested to influence the impression made upon others. These characteristics should therefore be considered during assessment as, in some instances, the client's difficulty in achieving successful outcomes from social interactions may be more a reflection of personal characteristics rather than what he or she actually says or does.

The characteristics of the situation and relevant others

To complicate matters further, it must be borne in mind that judgements of social competency are also influenced by the characteristics of the person making the judgement, other persons involved in the interaction and the situation involved. Given so many potential variables, it is not surprising to find that different responses are required for interactions with different people in different social situations. In any social interaction, one must take all these variables into account when selecting the most appropriate response (McFall, 1982). The final judgement regarding competency of the performance is also influenced by the characteristics of the judge, such as age, sex, culture, attitudes and knowledge about the interaction. When a therapist is required to assess a client's social performance, all these sources of influence should be considered, in addition to the actual behaviours engaged in by the client. Intervention may be more appropriately geared to alterations in situational aspects or the behaviour of other people with whom the client interacts, rather than changing the client's behaviour *per se*. Hence, it is important for the assessor to identify the type and nature of interactions with which the client must deal and the specific behaviours or skills that the client needs for adequate social functioning. Similarly, the clinician must be aware of the characteristics and responses of relevant people with whom the client interacts, in order to determine whether unrealistic expectations, faulty perception or inappropriate responding on the part of other people are contributing to the client's social difficulties. In particular, attention should be paid to ethnic and cultural factors that may have a bearing on the client's problems. Overall, considerable attention must be paid during assessment to the very many factors that determine whether a client experiences social success, over and above that he/she actually says and does.

Environmental contingencies

Social behaviour, as with any other aspect of human behaviour, is very much determined by antecedent and consequential contingencies within the individual's environment. If a social learning analysis (Bandura, 1977a) is applied to interpersonal behaviour, it can be seen as highly influenced by the modelling, prompting, reinforcement and punishment of others. When a client presents with problems of social competence, these factors must be taken into account, as there is little point in spending considerable time teaching social skills or reducing social anxiety if environmental influences are still operating to maintain inappropriate social responding. Poor social functioning may result from either a failure to learn to respond appropriately or from the acquisition of inappropriate response repertoires. In both instances, the individual's learning history is a contributory factor to the present difficulties. Current, relevant environmental contingencies or sources of modelling should be investigated during assessment, as successful intervention is likely to require changes to these factors. It may also be important to create new learning experiences for the client within his/her natural environment to increase or maintain appropriate responding and to reduce inappropriate social behaviour. This will require manipulation of antecedents (including modelling and prompting by others) and consequences within the client's day-to-day life. To some extent, information about factors that are currently maintaining the client's social problems can be obtained from interview with the client or relevant others. Ideally however, some degree of direct behavioural observation is needed to accurately identify these variables.

Social networks and social contacts

Obviously, the client's social network and range of social contacts may influence his/her social functioning. The opportunity to interact with family members, workmates and other people in recreational settings is likely to affect the individual's skill in interacting with others. Where opportunities are few, skill deficits may reflect a lack of practice, the chance to learn from others and/or confidence in the ability to deal with the situation. Intervention in such cases may require attempts to encourage clients to enter new social groups and to create opportunities for social interaction. The assessment of social networks is therefore important and may also identify resources, in the form of people within the client's social support system, who could be used in the therapy process to facilitate generalisation and maintenance of behaviour change.

A three-tier approach to the assessment of social problems

The approach taken to the assessment of interpersonal problems will depend upon what is already known about the client's social difficulties. In some instances, the first step is to establish whether a social problem exists. In others, the client is either self-referred or is referred by someone else specifically in relation to interpersonal problems. Let us assume for the purposes of this chapter that the client is aware of and acknowledges some form of interpersonal difficulty. Table 5.3 outlines a three-tier approach to the assessment of social difficulty. This structure may facilitate a hypothesis-testing approach to enable the assessor to clarify the nature of the client's presenting problems and to identify targets for intervention. It is important to point out that there are so many variables that influence social functioning that a complex model of determining factors comes to look like a spider's web. The three-tier model presented here is not designed to be a comprehensive model of social difficulty. Rather, it reflects the increase in complexity of assessment that can be used to test out hypotheses as to why a client is experiencing social problems.

At the first level, the assessor explores whether a problem exists in relation to frequency or response probability, the client's subjective report of negative emotion, or in terms of negative outcomes (e.g. lack of friends, failure to succeed in job interviews) in certain social situations. At this stage, and throughout the assessment process, a combination of self-report, other report and direct behavioural observation is needed. A variety of specific instruments may be used in addition to the behavioural interview. These will be discussed shortly. At the second level of the assessment process, the assessor begins to search for broad explanations as to the main presenting problems. Obviously, at each stage of assessment, more than one problem area may be identified and these may be interrelated. For example, at Level 1 a client could present with all three main problem areas, either alone or in any combination. The area then explored at Level 2 would depend on the findings at Level 1. For example, low frequency of a specific social behaviour could reflect deliberate avoidance on the part of the client or a lack of opportunity to engage in the activity. Similarly, negative outcomes could reflect an inadequate performance on the part of the client or unrealistic expectations of others. The nature of any negative emotions concerning the social situation concerned

Table 5.3: *A three-tier approach to the assessment of social difficulty*

Level 1: Is there a problem in one of these three main areas?	Low frequency or response probability		Subjective report of negative emotion	Negative outcomes	
Level 2: If so, what is the general area of the problem? (Clarification)	Lack of opportunity	Avoidance	Nature of negative emotion, e.g. anxiety, fear, anger	Characteristics of others + task demands e.g. excessive expectation, excessive task difficulty. Inappropriate response of others	Selection of inappropriate response or poor performance of appropriate strategies as judged by others
Level 3: Detailed assessment of causal factors	*Personal characteristics* Age, sex, physical appearance, dress, relevant psychopathology e.g. depression, *schizophrenia* Learning history	*Environmental factors* Opportunity Social networks, social support, modelling, prompting and reinforcement by other. Consequences of individual's behaviour	*Characteristics of social situation* — frequency — duration — where, when — who with — task demands — aims of participants	*Emotion* Motoric Cognitive Physiological Other cognitive determinants Attitudes Beliefs	*Skill repertoire* *Motoric* — basic + complex skill performance *Cognitive* — Social — perceptual Social problem-solving Self-monitoring Self-instructions Challenging of negative thoughts

also requires clarification.

Similarly, the findings at Levels 1 and 2 influence the area of assessment performed at Level 3. For example, if no evidence of negative affect was evident at Levels 1 or 2, then a detailed assessment of emotion would not be performed at Level 3. Similarly, if the client's responding was judged to be adequate at Level 2, then there would be little point in conducting a detailed assessment of specific social skills at Level 3. The information obtained at Level 3 should then enable the assessor to design an individually tailored intervention programme that tackles aetiological factors relating to the individual, his or her environment and others with whom he or she interacts.

Before discussing techniques for the collection of information, it is important to mention the role of certain forms of psychopathology in social-skills deficits. For example, individuals who suffer from schizophrenic disorders frequently exhibit inadequacies in social responding (Wallace, Nelson, Liberman, Aitchison, Lukoff, Elder & Ferris, 1980) and may experience extremely bizarre cognitive distortions with regard to their social relationships. Many clients suffering from depressive disorders are also suggested to exhibit deficiencies in social-skill performance (Libet & Lewinsohn, 1973). The cause-and-effect relationships between social skills and these forms of psychopathology are far from clear (Shepherd, 1983a). The possibility of schizophrenic and depressive symptomatology, however, obviously must be borne in mind when assessing a client with interpersonal difficulty. For example, if assessment reveals that the client reports a multitude of negative responses from others and assessment of other information sources reveals that this is not the case, the question of paranoid delusions may arise. It is beyond the scope of this chapter to explore fully the relevance of various forms of psychopathology to social functioning, but the assessor must at least be aware of its import.

Specific assessment measures

Several instruments are available to facilitate assessment at Levels 1 and 2 of the three-tier approach. The 'social situations questionnaire' (Bryant & Trower, 1974) for example, gives measures of degree of difficulty in terms of anxiety or discomfort, and frequency of participation in various social events. The 'Gambrill and Richey (1975) assertion inventory' measures the degree of discomfort and response probability, but is restricted to a range of assertive behaviours. The 'Watson and Friend (1969) social avoidance and distress scale ' (SAD) is also useful. This self-report questionnaire assesses the client's tendency to avoid and escape from social interactions and the degree of distress experienced during such interactions. The psychometric properties in terms of reliability and validity are acceptable but the majority of research has been conducted with college students rather than clinical populations, which somewhat limits its appropriateness to clinical practice. Some psychometric data is available for the Gambrill and Richey scale, but such information appears to be lacking for the Bryant and Trower instrument.

A more in-depth assessment of the type of situations that result in avoidance or distress can be obtained from the 'Richardson and Tasto (1976) social anxiety inventory'. This incorporates 105 items derived from hierarchies of socially anxious clients. It provides seven distinct fear factors; fear of disapproval or negative evaluation, social assertiveness and visibility; confrontation and anger expression, heterosexual contact, intimacy and interpersonal warmth, conflict with or rejection by parents and interpersonal loss. Curran, Corriveau, Monti & Hagerman (1980) provide psychometric data on Richardson and Tasto's social anxiety inventory obtained from a large group of psychiatric patients.

Whereas questionnaires of the type described can be used to assess response probability and subjective distress in social situations, the assessment of negative outcomes is dependent to a large extent on interviews with the client and relevant others. The use of a diary or self-monitoring sheet such as that shown in Table 5.4 may be helpful in identifying problem situations and providing information relating to relevant emotions and cognitions. The antecedent stimuli and consequences of the client's responding may also be elucidated.

Several specific assessment measures may also be used in relation to Level 3 factors. The assessment of microskills can be achieved in several ways, but the most commonly used technique involves role-played situations that are subject to the rating of specific behaviours and global judgements of performance by an independent observer. Ratings may be carried out from either live or from videotaped role-plays. The most well-known method is the 'behavioural assertiveness test' (revised) (Eisler, Hersen, Miller & Blanchard, 1975). The internal consistency and interobserver

Table 5.4: *Self-recording of target situation.*
Definition of target situation

Name:

Date	Time	Where are you?	Who with?	What do you do?	What happens next?	What emotions do you feel?		What were your thoughts?	
						Before?	After?	Before?	After?

reliability are reportedly good (Eisler *et al.*, 1975; Bellack, Hersen & Turner, 1978) but Bellack *et al.* raise questions as to the validity of role-play as being representative of real-life behaviour. This point should be borne in mind when using role-play assessment. Trower, Bryant and Argyle (1978) also provide a useful method of rating specific behaviours, but the psychometric properties are yet to be investigated. This method takes 29 social skills ranging from very specific microskills to complex response strategies (e.g. assertive routines). Ratings of performance are based on the subjective judgement of the observer, assisted by rating descriptors.

The 'Lowe and Cautela (1978) social performance survey schedule' is also useful in assessing general social performance and specific social-skill areas. It can be used either as a self-report or 'other'-report instrument and involves a list of 100 items covering a broad range of social interaction behaviours. A positive score composed of desirable responses can be determined separately from a negative score concerning undesirable social behaviours. Micro- and macroskill areas are covered and ratings are made according to probability of occurrence. Test–retest reliability is reportedly good, and its validity has been supported in several studies (Lowe, 1982, 1985; Miller & Funabiki, 1984).

The development of assessment devices for social-cognitive skills and maladaptive cognitions has received less attention. Several methods exist for exploring the client's ability in the area of social perception, such as the 'social interpretation task' (Archer & Akert, 1977) or the 'profile of nonverbal sensitivities' (Rosenthal, Hall, DiMatteo, Rogers & Archer, 1979). In practice, however, these methods are more designed to fit the needs of research programmes rather than clinical assessment (Arkowitz, 1981).

Most of the research into assessment of social problem-solving ability has focused on children but the 'means–ends problem-solving test' (Platt & Spivack, 1975) is one measure that may be useful with adults. Unfortunately, its psychometric properties appear to be weak (Butler & Meichenbaum, 1981), which may therefore limit its value.

The assessment of maladaptive cognitions in the determination of social difficulty is also in its infancy. The 'irrational beliefs test' (Alden & Safran, 1978) may be a useful start. The 'Watson and Friend (1969) fear of negative evaluation' (FNE) may also be helpful in that it considers the client's concern, apprehension and worry about the way others evaluate him/her.

The behavioural interview

The behavioural interview outlined in this chapter is designed to follow the three-tier approach to assessment of interpersonal problems. The initial phase determines whether a problem does exist for the client, corresponding to Level 1 of the assessment approach. This phase considers whether the problem relates to insufficient frequency of interaction with certain people, whether the client is experiencing discomfort during interactions and/or is failing to achieve successful outcomes from specific situations. Generally, the interviewer will have some prior knowledge from referring agencies or the client him/herself as to the broad category of the problem. For example, it may already be known that the client is complaining of lack of girl/boyfriends or is having trouble obtaining work through job interviews.

Subsequent sections of the interview then proceed to investigate the exact nature and determinants of the problem. Each section explores a different aspect of social dysfunction. The interviewer may find it useful to select certain sections rather than others, using a logical, hypothesis-testing model, rather than exploring all areas in depth.

The interview format in the initial stages of the interview must vary somewhat according to what is already known about the client, whether self- or other-referred and whether he or she acknowledges that a social problem exists. This latter point is important, as some clients may be oblivious to the existence of social difficulty and the complainant may be someone else in the client's life (e.g. referring nurse or spouse of a schizophrenic client). Alternatively, a social problem may be suspected secondary to some other presenting disorder, such as depression or alcohol abuse. Some general questions are suggested here, but the interviewer will need to use discretion and ingenuity in these early stages.

Introduction

> How do you feel you get on with people generally? Are there any aspects of your social life you would like to change? Has anybody ever commented that you have difficulty getting on with others . . . with any particular people . . . or in any particular situations?

Quantity of social interaction

> Are you satisfied with the amount of time you spend with other people — at work, at home, with your family/partner, socially, with boy/girlfriends (*if relevant*)?
> How much time do you spend, roughly, with people in each of these situations?
> How much of this time is actually spent talking with others?
> Do you take part in any activities with them?

At this point it is often helpful to ask the client to describe a typical weekday and weekend, in terms of contact with others. It is also important to bear in mind that some clients may be content with a low frequency of certain types of interaction and may not view this as a problem area. This point should be respected in programme planning.

> Do you have any opportunities to meet new people and make new friends? If not, why not? Would you prefer to have more contact with others?

Quality of social interaction/adverse outcomes

> Which people do you get on particularly well with? Are there any people in particular with whom you have difficulty? Can you describe what tends to happen here? What tends to go wrong?
> Are there any particular situations in which things don't turn out the way you would like them to?
> What tends to happen?
> How would you like things to work out in these situations?
> Are you aware of anything that you are doing or not doing that may be contributing to the problem?
> Do you have any close friendships? With whom?
> Are you able to confide your personal thoughts and feelings with anyone? Who are these?

Discomfort and/or avoidance

> Are there any social situations or people with whom you feel particularly uncomfortable or anxious (*or angry, if relevant*)?
> Can you describe these feelings a bit more?

The aim here is to identify the type of emotions experienced. In-depth assessment of negative emotions may then be conducted in the third level component of the assessment process:

> Do you tend to avoid situations that make you feel this way?
> Do you try to get out of the situation as quickly as possible?

Historical aspects and social development

Assuming that some general area of social problem is identified by this stage, the interviewer may then explore developmental aspects of the client's social functioning:

Can you tell me how long you have found (*the particular situation*) difficult?

Has it always been a problem?

What about when you were a child . . . did you have many friends?

Did you have any very close friendships?

As an adolescent, how did you get on with other kids at school?

Did you go out with your friends as a teenager? To what type of activities did you go?

If the difficulties relate to heterosexual relationships, the client's dating history should be explored at this point.

Clarification of the problem situation

Once it has been established that the client is experiencing interpersonal problems, the subsequent direction of the interview is determined to a large extent by the broad category of the problem. Fortunately, some common question areas can be identified, independent of the broad category, which can be used to specify the problem behaviour and identify antecedent and consequences, which may be maintaining the problem behaviour. The following questions may be useful in achieving these goals:

Can you describe a recent example of when (the problem) occurred? Where, when, with whom, what happened next?

Can you identify the type of situations in which the problem occurs?

With whom exactly? How often?

For how long has this been a problem to you?

Can you describe exactly what you do in these situations? (*Try to elicit the chain of behaviours the client engages in.*)

How do others respond? What do they say/do?

Are there any occasions when the problem does not occur? When, where and with whom?

Identification of relevant parameters of problem situation(s)

The interviewer progresses to identify the relevant parameters of the problem situation.

Do you find that you react differently or that the outcome is

different according to the number of people involved or with the age, sex, or status of other people involved, or with their personal qualities, such as whether they are talkative or serious?
Does your reaction differ according to how well you know the person or with the nature of the event, such as whether you're at a party, at lunch or at work?
Does the problem depend on what you are trying to do, for example, asking a favour, starting a conversation, giving a compliment, making a criticism, introducing people to each other or saying 'no' to a request?
Do you find the problem is reduced if any particular person is in the situation with you?

Clarification of social anxiety, or maladaptive cognitions

If it becomes evident that feelings of anxiety or discomfort are experienced in certain social situations, this area requires further exploration. Similarly, it is important to check out whether the client's responding is influenced by maladaptive cognitions. As mentioned earlier, both these factors may result in social-skill inhibition and/or avoidance of certain situations.

Physiological reactions

How exactly do you feel in the difficult situations?
What happens to you physically, e.g. racing heart, perspiration, blushing, difficulty in breathing or overbreathing, shaking limbs?

Cognitive aspects

What are you thinking to yourself before you go into the situation? What do you think or say to yourself once you're in it? How about afterwards?

Overt behavioural aspects

What exactly do you do beforehand . . . in the situation . . . afterwards? What do you say to the other person?

Where social anxiety is deemed to be a problem for the client, subsequent assessment sessions may then proceed to generate a hierarchy of social situations. This may then provide a basis for desensitisation procedures in combination with therapeutic input to deal with other contributing factors.

Clarification of social-skill usage

It is extremely difficult to obtain a good indication of social-skill usage from the behavioural interview part of the assessment for several reasons. First, although direct observation of the client by the assessor during interview may provide some information with regard to basic social-skill use (e.g. eye contact or posture), the situational specificity of behaviour must bring the validity of the information into question. In other words, the way the client responds to the interviewer in a clinical setting is not necessarily representative of the way the client responds in the naturalistic, problem situation. This criticism may also be applied to role-play assessment methods (Bellack, Hersen & Turner, 1978). Second, the client is not necessarily aware of his/her social-skill deficits and direct questioning about skill usage is not always useful, as many people underestimate or overestimate their own social-skills ability (Youngren & Lewinsohn, 1980). Despite these limitations, it is suggested that some provisional social-skill data can be obtained during the behavioural interview. This can then be checked out against reports from relevant others, self-monitoring by the client or direct behavioural observation in the naturalistic situation. The list of social-skill areas in Table 5.1 may facilitate the assessment in terms of direct observation by the assessor. Ideally, however, a much more detailed assessment of social skills should be performed, such as that outlined by Trower, Bryant and Argyle (1978).

Identification of other determinants of interpersonal problems

As mentioned previously, it is also important for the assessor to determine the degree to which it is the response of others or some characteristic of the client, other than what he/she says and does in the social interaction, which is accounting for an adverse outcome from social situations. Factors such as the client's personal appearance and dress should therefore be considered during interview. Similarly, information regarding the characteristics of other people involved in the social situations of concern may be beneficial to the assessment process.

Concluding the interview

In the final phase of the interview, it is important to investigate the types of methods that the client has already tried as a means of tackling the problem. Obviously, as social problems are likely to present in conjunction with other difficulties, such as depression, exploration of other areas will also be necessary. As with any other of the topics discussed in this book, it is also emphasised that additional data should be obtained from self-report questionnaires, diaries, self-monitoring, information from relevant others and direct behavioural observation. Such information, combined with data from the behavioural interview, should facilitate the generation of an individually tailored behaviour-therapy programme.

Treatment of interpersonal problems

A variety of techniques have been applied to the remediation of interpersonal problems. These have differed in terms of the focus of intervention, such as the level of skill complexity and the degree of incorporation of cognitive versus overt behavioural-skills training. Terms such as 'structured learning therapy' (Goldstein, 1973), 'personal effectiveness training' (Liberman, King, De Risi & McCann, 1975), 'assertion training' (Wolpe & Lazarus, 1966) and 'social-skills training' (Hersen & Bellack, 1976) abound in the literature. Despite variation in focus and content of intervention, these approaches have in common the aim to teach specific skills by means of instructions, discussion, modelling, role-play/practice, feedback and homework assignments. Superimposed upon this basic core of intervention are various other approaches, such as restructuring of maladaptive cognitions, teaching of social-perception skills and social problem-solving skills and anxiety-management techniques.

The variation in content of intervention programmes and the widely differing characteristics of persons with whom the approaches have been applied, makes it difficult to draw general conclusions about the effectiveness of treatment. Social-enhancement programmes have been applied with numerous client groups including psychiatric inpatients (Wallace, Nelson, Liberman, Aitchison, Lukoff, Elder & Ferris, 1980), psychiatric outpatients (Marzillier, Lambert & Kellet, 1976), depressed clients (Nezu, 1986), alcohol abusers (Van Hasselt, Hersen & Milliones, 1978) and socially anxious persons (Van Dam-Baggen & Kraaimaat, 1986), to mention just a few. Review papers tend to be cautiously optimistic (Scott, Himadi & Keane, 1983; Shepherd, 1983b).

Shepherd points out, however, that numerous methodological problems exist in most research studies conducted to date. Assessment of maintenance and generalisation to the client's natural environment is rarely adequate and the evaluation measures used, if any, are frequently of questionable reliability and validity and tend to rely on self-report rather than objective evidence or other person's report. Shepherd concludes that the more rigorous the assessment of generalisation and maintenance, the less impressive the results of social-enhancement programmes become.

Rather than ending on a pessimistic note, perhaps it is important to look at why this might be the case and what could be done to rectify matters. First, it must be acknowledged that most research studies have used a package approach to treatment that pays little heed to the specific difficulties and causal factors for individual clients. It would seem sensible to suggest that intervention is most likely to be effective when individually tailored to remediate the problem areas of each client. Second, there has been a tendency amongst researchers to select clients for social-skills training or social-enhancement programmes based upon membership of some diagnostic group such as 'depressed', 'alcoholic', or 'schizophrenic'. Attempts are rarely made to determine whether or not each client actually does have difficulty in interpersonal situations. A danger exists, therefore, of clients being selected for treatment studies when no deficit exists in the skills being taught. A careful assessment would seem to be needed for each client to establish the existence of interpersonal problems and the nature and causes of such difficulties. This should then allow the design of intervention programmes that tackle relevant skills for each client and increase the probability of his/her overcoming the interpersonal problem of concern.

Finally, few programmes have paid adequate attention to methods of increasing generalisation and maintenance of treatment effects. Methods such as training within natural settings, incorporating relevant others from the client's environment into training sessions, using a wide range of trainers and ensuring that relevant skills are selected have all been suggested to be important means of enhancing generalisation (Goldstein, Sherman, Gershaw, Sprafkin & Glick, 1978). To date, very few research studies have succeeded in including those components into therapy. Furthermore, there has also been little attempt to facilitate maintenance of therapy, for example, by the use of booster sessions. Given the lack of attention to programming for generalisation and maintenance of treatment gains, it is perhaps not surprising to find relatively weak therapy effects. It is suggested here that closer attention to these issues is important if lasting improvements are to be obtained in clients' social functioning.

6
Assessment of Sexual Dysfunction

Introduction

Sexual dysfunction, as with any other human-behaviour problem may be subjected to a detailed behavioural analysis. This enables the practitioner to identify the nature of the presenting dysfunction and the antecedents and consequences that are currently maintaining the problem. The behaviour itself must be understood in terms of the physiological, cognitive and overt behavioural components. The determinants of sexual behaviour, however, are enormously complex and the assessor needs a thorough understanding of the anatomical, physiological, biochemical and psychosocial factors involved. Such information is given in detail in texts such as Kaplan (1974) and Masters & Johnson (1966).

Phases of sexual responding

Sexual responding may be classified into three separate phases in both the male and the female, namely the arousal phase, the orgasm phase and resolution. In the male, arousal typically involves erection of the penis, tightening of the scrotal sac, raising of the testicles within the scrotum and general bodily reactions such as increased muscle tension, blood pressure, heart rate and respiration rate. In the female, a similar vasocongestive response occurs during sexual arousal causing vaginal lubrication, vaginal lengthening and formation of the orgasmic platform around the base of the vagina. Some clitoral engorgement may also occur and the labia may change in colour. Similar general body responses occur during this phase to those found in the male. During the orgasm phase for the male, two separate components can be identified — emission and expulsion. Emission involves contraction of the internal sex organs as semen is placed at the entrance to the urethra. This is then followed by expulsion, in which rhythmic contractions of the penile urethra and muscles at the base of the penis occur at around 0.8 sec intervals, forcing ejaculate from the penis. In the woman, the orgasm phase involves similar rhythmic contractions, but of the orgasmic platform. This is usually preceeded by a retraction of the clitoris under the clitoral hood.

Finally, the resolution phase occurs which, in the male, involves a refractory period where gradual detumescence occurs and little response results from further sexual stimulation. The length of this period varies according to the individual and the age of the man involved. Females typically have a much briefer resolution phase, but general detumescence occurs in much the same way as for the male.

Definition of terms

Before considering the aetiological factors involved in different types of sexual dysfunction, it is first helpful to have a knowledge of terminology and the characteristics of various sexual dysfunctions. Given the complex nature of human sexual behaviour, it is not surprising to find a variety of sexual dysfunctions, each of which may be associated with a complex range of determinants. Generally, sexual problems can be viewed as a failure of either the arousal and/or orgasm component of the sexual response. The aim of the assessor is therefore to identify the nature of the presenting problem and to clarify the determinants from both an historical and current perspective.

The APA, DSM-III-R (1987) criteria for a diagnosis of a sexual dysfunction require that the problem cannot be attributed entirely to organic factors, an Axis I mental disorder such as a major depression or due to inadequate sexual stimulation. The various types of sexual dysfunctions are categorised into disorders of sexual desire, orgasm and sexual pain.

Hypoactive sexual desire disorder

This is defined by DSM-III-R as:

> persistently or recurrently deficient or absent sexual fantasies and desire for sexual activity. The judgment of deficiency or absence is made by the clinician, taking into account factors that affect sexual functioning, such as age, sex and the context of the person's life.
>
> (APA, DSM-III-R, 1987, p. 293)

Sexual aversion disorder

This term is defined by DSM-III-R as 'persistent or recurrent extreme aversion to, and avoidance of, all or almost all, genital sexual contact with a sexual partner' (APA, DSM-III-R, 1987, p. 293).

Male erectile disorder

According to DSM-III-R this term is applied to either:

> (1) persistent or recurrent partial or complete failure in a male to attain or maintain erection until completion of the sexual activity or (2) persistent or recurrent lack of a subjective sense of sexual excitement and pleasure in a male during sexual activity.
>
> (APA, DSM-III-R, 1987, p. 294)

This term has been referred to elsewhere in the literature as erectile failure, erectile difficulty and impotence.

Female sexual arousal disorder

The classification is used in relation to:

> (1) persistent or recurrent partial or complete failure to attain or maintain the lubrication–swelling response of sexual excitement until completion of the sexual activity or (2) persistent or recurrent lack of a subjective sense of sexual excitement and pleasure in a female during sexual activity.
>
> (APA, DSM-III-R, 1987, p. 294)

Inhibited female orgasm

This term is applied to the 'persistent or recurrent delay in, or absence of, orgasm in a female following a normal sexual excitement phase during sexual activity that the clinician judges to be adequate in focus, intensity and duration' (APA, DSM-III-R, 1987, p. 294). It is pointed out that some women are able to experience orgasm during noncoital clitoral stimulation but are unable to experience it during coitus in the absence of manual clitoral stimulation. The point is made that this is a relatively normal, state of affairs.

Inhibited male orgasm

This refers to:

> persistent or recurrent delay in, or absence of, orgasm in the male following a normal sexual excitement phase during sexual activity that the clinician, taking into account the person's age, judges to be adequate in focus, intensity, and duration. This failure to achieve orgasm is usually restricted to an inability to reach orgasm in the vagina, with orgasm possible with other types of stimulation such as masturbation.
>
> (APA, DSM-III-R, 1987, p. 295)

The terms 'delayed' or 'retarded' ejaculation are also widely used in practice.

Premature ejaculation

DSM-III-R applies this term in relation to:

> persistent or recurrent ejaculation with minimal sexual stimulation or before, upon, or shortly after penetration and before the person wishes it. The clinician must take into account factors that affect duration of the excitement phase, such as age, novelty of the sexual partner or situation, and frequency of sexual activity.
>
> (APA, DSM-III-R, 1987, p. 295)

Dyspareunia

This refers to 'recurrent and persistent genital pain in either a male or a female before, during or after sexual intercourse'. The condition must not be caused exclusively by a physical disorder and is not due to lack of lubrication or vaginismus (APA, DSM-III-R, 1987, p. 295).

Vaginismus

Vaginismus refers to the 'recurrent and persistent involuntary spasm of the musculature of the outer third of the vagina that interferes with coitus' (APA, DSM-III-R, 1987, p. 295).

Kaplan (1974) points out that, in severe cases, this may also involve the rectal and gluteus leg muscles. The response may be triggered by real, imagined or anticipated attempts at penetration of the vagina. The spasms produced frequently result in painful intercourse and this in turn creates further tension and anxiety, making painful intercourse even more likely. A vicious cycle may therefore become established.

In relation to all types of sexual dysfunction, DSM-III-R emphasises that the problem can be either primary, occurring under all situations, or secondary, occurring in some circumstances and not others.

Biological determinants of sexual dysfunction

Human sexual behaviour is determined by a host of biological, environmental and psychological influences. As a result, there are numerous explanations for why the process of sexual responding may break down. The assessor needs a sound understanding of these determinants in order to identify areas that may be tackled during the therapy process. Although the focus here is on behavioural assessment and intervention, a competent knowledge of biological aspects is particularly important for those working with sexually dysfunctional clients.

The responses of erection, ejaculation and lubrication may result from reflex mechanisms triggered by physical stimulation of the genitals. These operate through the spinal cord and lower brain stem, but are typically modified and controlled by higher cortical activity. Hence, activity in either of these higher or lower neural pathways may influence the arousal or orgasm components. Overall, however, a complex interaction of physical stimulation and cognitive activity is important in determining how a person responds sexually. In relation to lower neural control, it is important to note that the arousal and orgasm phases are controlled by separate neural pathways, the arousal phase being controlled by local parasympathetic networks and the orgasm phase by sympathetic pathways. This explains why, for some clients, only the arousal phase is disturbed but the orgasm phase may be adequate. With other clients, arousal may occur but the orgasm component is not achieved and in some instances, both arousal and orgasm may be affected. Drugs, illnesses and biological processes, which differentially affect parasympathetic and sympathetic pathways, may produce different influences on the arousal and orgasm components of sexual functioning.

Traditionally, it has been held that certain characteristics of sexual responding can be identified that suggest organic versus psychosocial causes for sexual dysfunction. With male clients, for example, the selective occurence of erection or orgasm rather than total absence has frequently been proposed to imply a psychosocial aetiology, whereas total absence of these responses may be more indicative of an organic aetiology. Similarly, an organic cause for ejaculatory failure is often assumed to be unlikely if the male can masturbate to orgasm but cannot achieve ejaculation during coitus. Freund and Blanchard (1981), however, caution as to drawing conclusions concerning organic versus psychosocial aetiology on the basis of such simplistic criteria. These authors point out that an organic basis should not be excluded when intermittent sexual functioning is present. Hence, the presence of nocturnal penile tumescence should not necessarily be taken as definite evidence against the involvement of organic factors in erectile failure. Similarly, the ability to masturbate to orgasm or achieve an erection during masturbation should not be taken as conclusive evidence against organic involvement in orgasmic dysfunction or erectile failure. Given the enormous complexity of the biological systems involved in sexual behaviour, it is strongly suggested that the task of excluding organic variables is left to suitably qualified medical practitioners. Nevertheless, the assessor should acquire an adequate knowledge of the numerous organic determinants of sexual dysfunction.

Illness

A variety of diseases and illnesses may impair sexual responding. In some instances, such effects may be direct, for example, interference in the hormonal, vascular or neural systems that regulate sexual responding or physical damage to the sex organs. In others, the impairment may be an indirect result of illness or injury. The individual may be capable theoretically of adequate sexual responding, but fails to do so. For example, avoidance of sexual activity may be related to fear of further injury such as may be found following myocardial infarction. Alternatively, avoidance of sex may serve to prevent pain to other body parts that may result from sexual activity, as may be the case for persons suffering from chronic back pain or arthritis. Many serious illnesses also result in a reduction in sexual desire because of general feelings of ill health and fatigue. Furthermore, some illnesses cause severe disfigurement of the body and may cause the client to develop concerns as to their physical attractiveness to their partner. These issues are highlighted by Anderson and Wolf (1986) in an interesting paper that discusses the psychological consequences of serious illness that may interfere with sexual functioning.

Even where there is direct involvement of an illness in sexual difficulties, the degree of impairment may exceed that caused specifically by the illness. For example, Whitehead, Klyde, Zussman, Wayne, Shinbach and Davis (1983) suggest that a significant contribution to erectile failure amongst men with diabetes mellitus is made from the adverse psychological experiences of the disorder, such as anxiety, depression, fear and lethargy. Diabetes mellitus is thought to impair erectile responding in some males due to damage to the peripheral nerves and small blood vessels caused by chronic, high blood-glucose levels (Anderson & Wolf, 1986). It seems likely, however, that erectile problems are exacerbated by the adverse psychological consequences of the condition.

Detailed descriptions of the major physical conditions that affect sexual responding are available in Jehu (1979) and Kaplan (1974). This chapter provides only a brief outline of the major neural, vascular and endocrine disorders that may result in sexual problems. Basically, any illness or injury that impairs the neural, vascular or endocrine systems that control the various aspects of sexual responding may result in sexual dysfunction. The nature of the problem, whether it be in the arousal or in the orgasm phase, will depend on the physiological stage affected.

Neural impairment. In the case of neurological impairment, the type of sexual problem produced will depend on the location and extent of the lesion. Sexual dysfunction resulting from neural impairment at a cortical level is relatively rare, but certain lesions within the hypothalamus or limbic system may interfere with sexual functioning (Kaplan, 1974). Neurological damage within the spinal cord is a more frequent cause of sexual problems, albeit still a relatively rare phenomenon. Such damage may result from accidents, surgical procedures, tumours, inflamation, multiple sclerosis, other degenerative diseases and congenital defects (e.g. spina bifida). The type of sexual problems produced will depend on the location of the lesion, which determines the type of neural pathways affected. Jehu (1979) proposes that any lesion that affects any of the following may impair sexual responding:

1. The afferent nerves carrying sensory input to the spinal centres,
2. These centres and their ascending and descending fibres to and from the brain,
3. The efferent autonomic and motor nerves that trigger off and control the sexual responses,
4. The relevant parts of the brain itself. (p. 23)

The majority of research into the effect of illness and drugs upon sexual responding has been carried out with males. Hence, discussion here will refer primarily to the effect upon erectile functioning and ejaculation.

Depending on the location and extent of the lesion, the effect may be to impair either the erectile response, the ejaculation component or both. The location of the lesion may also determine the type of stimulation to which the person is able to respond sexually. For example, if the neural lesion occurs above the sacral region of the spinal cord, the erectile response is usually maintained in response to tactile stimulation but not to other forms of stimulation such as fantasy, which involve higher cortical control via the thoracolumbar pathways. Alternatively, if the lesion occurs in the sacral region, erections may be possible through fantasy or visual stimulation and do not occur in response to tactile stimulation, which requires the sacral pathways to be intact (Jehu, 1979). Ejaculatory ability generally requires intact functioning of both the sacral and thoracolumbar regions. In practice, the effect on erectile and ejaculatory functioning will depend on the extent of the lesion and whether it is complete.

Diseases and injury to local neural pathways may also impair sexual responding. Diabetes mellitus is one example, with around 30 to 60 per cent of males with this condition experiencing erectile disorder (Jehu, 1979). In addition, some males with this condition may exhibit retrograde ejaculation in which semen is sent backwards into the bladder, resulting in dry ejaculation (Kaplan, 1974). The effects of diabetes mellitus on female sexual responding has been less well researched, and evidence concerning the effect on arousal and orgasm is conflicting (Anderson & Wolf, 1986). However, there is some suggestion that females with this condition are more prone to vaginal infection and dyspareunia, which may have a secondary effect on sexual activity (Krosnick & Podolsky, 1981).

Vascular diseases. If the local vasocongestive response is affected by an illness, then this is likely to impair erectile ability or the lubrication–swelling phase in women. Local thrombotic diseases are implicated here and diabetes mellitus has also been suggested to result in vascular deterioration in addition to neural impairment.

Hormonal/endocrine disorders. A range of tumours, congenital defects, infections and physical injuries may disrupt the hormonal system that influences sexual behaviour. The hypothalamic–pituitary–gonad system regulates the level of circulating sex hormones and may be interrupted at various stages, resulting in impairment of sexual arousal (Kaplan, 1974). Hypopituitarism, Cushing's syndrome, testicular tumours, ovarian tumours, castration, hepatic cirrhosis leading to testicular atrophy and certain congenital defects such as Klinefelter's syndrome are examples of disorders that may affect the endocrine system so as to impair sexual functioning.

The effect of menopause on women also deserves mention here. Although the effects are unclear, the reduced oestrogen levels that occur during menopause may cause some women to experience degenerative changes in the vagina, which becomes more prone to infection and inflammation. Impairment of lubrication is also evident for some women and both these conditions may result in painful intercourse (Jehu, 1979).

Genital impairment. Physical injury, inflammation or infection of the genital structures may interfere with sexual responding. Structural defects such as clitoral adhesions or poor episiotomies in women and excessively tight foreskins in males may inhibit satisfactory sex. Infections such as urethritis, cystitis and prostatitis are examples of the many infections that may also produce pain during intercourse (Masters & Johnson, 1970).

Drug effects

A wide range of chemical substances may interfere with sexual functioning, the exact nature of which will depend on the biological action of the drug involved. Any drug that affects the neural, endocrine or vascular systems involved in sexual functioning may impair sexual responding. The assessor therefore needs to pay particular attention to any substance used by the client, whether it be prescribed medication, illicit drugs or alcohol.

Sedatives. Sedative compounds such as alcohol or barbiturates are known to have a depressing effect on brain functioning, which may impair sexual functioning (Jehu, 1979). At low dosages, sedatives may have a disinhibitory effect that may enhance sexual arousal for some individuals. This is suggested to be a general disinhibitory effect and is not specific to sexual behaviour. At high doses, the general depressant effect on cortical functioning occurs and this may suppress the erectile response in males. With prolonged alcohol abuse, erectile failure may persist and is suggested to result from vascular and neural impairment, rather than from the depressant effect (Jehu, 1979).

Antihypertensives. Certain drugs that are used to control blood pressure may have an adverse effect on sexual functioning. In particular, beta-blocking agents are found to reduce erectile ability in some males, probably due to impairment of the parasympathetic pathways involved in the control of erections. Other forms of antihypertensives may also influence ejaculation and erectile ability. For example, guanethidine sulphate (ismelin), which is thought to prevent release of noradrenaline from the nerve endings (Silverstone & Turner, 1982), is suggested to interfere in both erectile and ejaculatory responding in over 50 per cent of males taking therapeutic dosages and in some instances, retrograde ejaculation may occur (Jehu, 1979).

Antipsychotic drugs. There is evidence to suggest that some drugs within the phenothiazine and butyrophenone groups and their derivatives may interfere with sexual functioning. Amongst the phenothiazines, thioridazine (mellaril) in particular has been noted to result in erectile difficulty, reduced ejaculate and retrograde ejaculation in some males (Kotin, Wilbert, Verburg & Soldinger, 1976). Within the butyrophenones, halperidol compounds have been reported to produce arousal and erectile problems in some instances (Kaplan, 1974).

Antidepressants. Both the monoamine reuptake inhibitors and the monoamine oxidase inhibitors may lead to partial erectile and ejaculatory problems for some males (Silverstone & Turner, 1982). Fortunately, the trycyclic antidepressants appear to have fewer sexual side effects (Kaplan, 1974).

Oral contraceptives. Evidence concerning the influence of oral contraceptives on sexual functioning is conflicting, but there is a suggestion that, for some women, the use of oral contraceptives may reduce sexual-arousal levels (Trimmer, 1978).

Ageing

The way in which people respond sexually changes over their life span. This must be taken into consideration when deciding whether a sexual problem is present or whether the change in response is merely a result of the ageing process. In the male, ageing is generally accompanied by an increase in the time taken to attain an erection and a greater time to regain an erection once it has been lost. The refractory period also typically increases and some subjective changes may be experienced, such as a reduction in the feeling of inevitability that is associated with the emission phase. Despite these changes, males are generally able to achieve erection and ejaculation from puberty throughout their life span.

Females also show changes in sexual responding with age, the most obvious change being a decline in the number of contractions during orgasm and a reduction in size of the orgasmic platform in later life. As with the male, women can generally continue to achieve orgasm throughout their lives. Menopause, however, may produce difficulties for some women, particularly if lubrication is reduced or takes longer to occur.

Psychosocial determinants of sexual dysfunction

Having outlined the major biological influences upon sexual responding, it is important to consider some of the psychosocial determinants. It must be stressed that, even when biological influences are found, these may be confounded by psychosocial factors that must also be tackled during the therapy phase.

Psychological state

Depression and fatigue are likely to inhibit arousal and make attainment of orgasm less likely. Anxiety may also exert an inhibitory effect and has traditionally been suggested to result in sexual dysfunction, particularly if the anxiety relates specifically to sexual activities (Masters & Johnson, 1970). This area is discussed in more detail in relation to cognitive factors.

Educational factors

A person's knowledge of sexual anatomy and sexual techniques has important applications for a successful sexual relationship. In particular, a knowledge of appropriate means of stimulating the partner is necessary and may account for a lack of arousal and/or orgasm for the partner. This area has been emphasised in relation to primary inhibitory female orgasm, in which education regarding masturbatory techniques has been a major focus of therapy (Heiman, LoPiccolo & LoPiccolo, 1976).

Attitudinal factors

A person's attitude towards various sexual activities and religious contraventions may have a considerable influence over the type of sexual activities they engage in and their response in terms of arousal and orgasm. Similarly, attitudes regarding sex roles during sex and expectancies regarding appropriate partner behaviour may be relevant. When considering this area, it is important to explore specific thoughts that the client experiences during different stages of sexual encounters. This may pinpoint maladaptive cognitions that are impairing sexual responsiveness.

Anxiety-related cognitions

In particular, maladaptive cognitions related to anxiety and fear may be important. Masters and Johnson (1970) place considerable emphasis on thoughts of fear of failure, 'spectatoring' or focusing on one's performance rather than on pleasure, and anticipation of pain or hurt.

Emotional reactions

Emotions such as anger, guilt, fear, disgust or shame may interfere with sexual functioning and may be triggered off during sexual interactions. In particular, it seems important to explore the clients' emotions and thoughts with regard to their partner during sex — do they feel physical attraction for each other, do they like/dislike each other, would they prefer to be with someone else? The area of marital satisfaction becomes particularly important in that marital disharmony has been suggested to be associated with certain sexual problems such as secondary female orgasmic dysfunction. Whether this is a cause or effect relationship, however, remains to be clarified (McGovern, Stewart & LoPiccolo, 1975).

Sexual preference

The client's sexual preferences in terms of degree of arousal to heterosexual or homosexual stimuli may influence their response to their partner's stimulation. Similarly, erotic preferences in terms of anomalous stimuli should be considered, e.g. voyeurism, sadism, transvestism (Freund & Blanchard, 1981).

Fantasy ability

Fantasy has been suggested to be an important means of achieving and enhancing sexual arousal and may be lacking with some individuals (Heiman, LoPiccolo & LoPiccolo, 1976). This area requires exploration in that training in the use of fantasy may be used during therapy to increase arousal levels.

Misinterpretation of stimulation and response

It is possible that for some people, the attention, reception, perception and interpretation process for incoming sexual stimuli may be faulty. For example, a person may fail to attend to the cues available and be unaware of his or her signs of arousal. Alternatively, arousal cues may be misinterpreted as an aversive feeling rather than pleasurable, or may be interpreted as a sign of anxiety rather than sexual arousal. Each of these areas should be explored for a thorough assessment.

Sexual skills

The sexual skills of both members of a sexual partnership may influence the success of the relationship. This involves two primary areas — physical-stimulation skills and communication skills. Each person needs to be able to stimulate their partner appropriately and to achieve positions during sex from which they can obtain the greatest amount of arousal and pleasure themselves. From the communication perspective, the couple need to be able to initiate sexual interactions, to give feedback appropriately, to request certain activities and to turn down requests for sex in an acceptable manner. Each sexual encounter involves a complex series of interactions, each of which demands a range of social skills. Inappropriate communication by either member of the partnership may interfere with successful sexual responding (Spence, 1983).

Physical environment factors

A variety of external environmental factors may influence sexual responding. Lack of opportunity, lack of privacy or a cold, uncomfortable setting are typical examples of events that may be associated with an unsatisfactory sexual relationship, hence the need to consider such factors during assessment.

Life events

A wide range of life events need to be considered during the interview. In a sense this is a secondary level of assessment, in that life events may be the cause of various psychogenic factors that influence sexual responding. For example, the client's anxiety may be the result of a loss of employment, depression could be triggered by death of a family member, or fatigue could be the result of excessive demands at work.

Consequences of the sexual dysfunction

The majority of determinants discussed can be classified as antecedents of the problem behaviour in that they typically exist prior to the occurrence of the problem. Although such events, whether internal or external in nature, are crucial to the understanding of the problem, it is important that the consequences of the behaviour are not forgotten. For example, the response of both partners to the occurrence of the dysfunction must be considered, as they may be important in maintaining the difficulty.

General points regarding assessment

In most instances, clients presenting with sexual difficulties will be involved in a regular relationship with a partner. In such cases, it is important that both persons are involved in the assessment, as the difficulty generally relates to the way in which the couple interact together sexually rather than being any one person's problem. The presence of both members of the partnership has the advantage of maximising the amount of information provided. Inconsistency between the partners' report may provide useful information in itself. The assessor is also able to ask each person how they feel their partner would answer each question. This may highlight distortions of perception and misunderstandings if discrepancies are found.

There are no hard-and-fast rules as to the way in which information-gathering should proceed. In some instances, clients may be single or their partners may not be willing to participate in assessment of therapy. Generally, when couples are involved, assessment may include an interview with the couple together and then with each member of the partnership separately. Some clients may be threatened by either aspect of this interview procedure, and the assessor will need to tread cautiously in deciding which format to use. Interviewing clients with sexual difficulties requires considerable skill in enabling the clients to feel relaxed and trusting. Thus, the initial stages of client contact may be geared towards the development of an optimal therapist–client relationship from which the clients feel able to discuss and divulge sensitive, personal information. This may be facilitated by assuring the clients that such problems are not uncommon and that it is necessary to ask personal information in order to plan an effective treatment strategy. The clients also need to be assured as to the confidentiality of any information revealed to the assessor.

If members of the partnership are to be interviewed separately, it is debatable whether the interviewer should encourage clients to divulge information that they do not wish their partner to know. This may be avoided by stating at the outset of client contact that all information must be freely shared by the couple. Alternatively, the assessor may prefer to elicit such sensitive information, respecting each partner's right to confidentiality. This approach may produce problems if secrets between one partner and the assessor make the conduct of therapy difficult, for example, if the interviewer discovers that one member of the partnership is involved in a satisfactory sexual relationship with someone else, unknown to their partner. This may make therapy a questionable goal, particularly if one member does not wish to engage in therapy or does not desire to achieve a satisfactory relationship with the regular partner. The assessor may then need to convey to the couple that therapy is not possible, without divulging the exact reason why.

A couple of other general points with regard to interviewing should be mentioned here. It is important that, in interviewing the clients, the terminology used is understandable. This may require the use of some jargon and terms preferred by the clients, while trying to avoid terms that may shock them. There is a danger too of presenting questions in a way that leads clients to expect orgasm on every occasion or to see orgasm as an overvalued goal. The terms 'achieve', 'attain' and 'reach' should therefore be avoided in relation to orgasm.

Finally, it is suggested that clients seeking psychological

treatment for sexual disorders are asked to undergo an examination by a medical practitioner. It is important that any organically caused sexual disorders receive the appropriate medical intervention necessary for a successful outcome. In many instances, there may be secondary psychosocial factors that are exacerbating or maintaining the problem, in which case, a psychologically based intervention may be necessary in conjunction with a medical approach.

The behavioural interview

Identifying the nature of the problem

The first step in the assessment interview is to determine why the client is seeking help and to specify the presenting problem. The assessor needs to identify exactly what the client does overtly, how he or she responds physiologically and what thoughts and emotions are experienced in the cognitive domain. Wincze (1982) also suggests that sexual disorders be classified according to problems of sexual anxiety, sexual arousal and/or unsatisfactory orgasm. The content of therapy will obviously be influenced by the nature of the presenting problem and this type of categorisation may facilitate the selection of a treatment strategy. Some of the following suggested questions may help the assessor to specify the nature of the problem:

What do you see as being the problem?

What triggered you to seek therapy?

To whom is it a problem? What effect does the problem have on each of you?

Under what circumstances does the problem occur — when, with whom, in what locations?

Has it always been a problem or is it only problematic in certain circumstances? When is the problem NOT present?

Can you describe to me what typically happens in your sexual relationship at the moment?

How often do you try to have sex? Where would you usually be (*location*) and when would you try (*time of day, etc.*)? Who would make the first move? How is this done?

What do you/he/she say/do? What methods of foreplay do you use? For how long? What kind of foreplay do you enjoy? How often do you give/receive this? Do either of you have an orgasm during intercourse? How long after penetration begins?

What methods do you use to help you have an orgasm? Do you orgasm during intercourse, during petting, during self-pleasuring? What type of stimulation is needed? Are there any things your partner could do to help that he/she doesn't do now? How do feel emotionally during sex? What thoughts are going through your head at different stages? Do you become aroused physiologically (*e.g. erection in the male/lubrication in the female*)? Is this ever a problem to you?

Do you ever try to vary what you do before and during sex? In what way? Can you tell me how you would like your sexual relationship to be? How often would you like to have sex? How often would you expect to have an orgasm? What sexual activities would you like to engage in? Can you describe what you think good sex should be like?

How long would you like intercourse to last?

Generally, the aim of the assessor at this stage is to determine exactly what is going on during the clients' sexual encounters. It is important to identify the type of physical stimulation being given and received and to determine whether this is adequate to allow arousal/orgasm to occur. Information is also needed regarding how the client responds both cognitively and physiologically. The assessor needs to know which phases of the sexual response are non-problematic and the point at which difficulties occur. Most importantly, what must be identified is whether the problem is one of excess arousal/inadequate arousal or lack of orgasm despite an adequate arousal response. The roles of anxiety and depression also need to be explored, as discussed earlier in this chapter. (See also Chapters 2 and 3 for a detailed assessment format.)

Having determined the nature of the presenting problem, the assessor is then in a position to compare the client's current sexual functioning with what could be considered 'normal' sexual behaviour. This allows the practitioner to decide whether the problem is one of inadequate sexual functioning or unrealistic expectations. Later on in the interview, the role of each member of the partnership in contributing to the problem can be determined. For example, the inadequate response of one member may be the result of inadequate stimulation from the other rather than an inadequate degree of responding.

Identification of determinants

During this part of the interview, the assessor needs to separate out historical and current determinants of the problem. It is likely that the current sources of influence will be those that can be manipulated during therapy to produce behaviour change. Current influences can be classified into the antecedents (external and internal in nature) and consequences of behaviour. External antecedents refer to stimuli within the environment, such as the partner's touch or the sight of a naked body. Internal antecedents, on the other hand, refer to physiological or cognitive events within the client, such as a state of tiredness, menstruation occurring or specific thoughts experienced by the client. The consequences of the problem behaviour refer to internal or external events that typically occur after the client has exhibited the sexual dysfunction, for example, feelings of failure or negative comments from the partner.

The following interview guidelines are designed to elicit information regarding current and historical determinants of the sexual problem. The major emphasis should be on current influences, but the role of historic factors should not be ignored. These may be important in enabling the assessor to fully understand why the problem developed and the type of intervention required. Having obtained the necessary information, the practitioner must then organise it within a comprehensive framework as suggested above in order to develop a treatment strategy.

Relevant background factors

The following outline pinpoints some of the most likely life events that may have occurred and that may have a bearing on the clients' current difficulties. The assessor may find other relevant areas that should be covered with particular clients.

Age. To consider the influence on sexual behaviour.

Religious and moral influences.

Do you currently belong to a religious group? Is this a serious commitment? Does this influence your views about sex? Did religious beliefs influence your views about sex when you were a child or teenager?

What are your strong moral beliefs about sex or any sexual activities?

Cultural/ethnic influences.

Are there important beliefs in your culture about sex that might be relevant here? (*Explore sex roles, in particular, sexual taboos, etc.*)

Parental influences

What kind of attitudes did your parents have towards sex? Was sex discussed in the home? Did your parents give you any education about sex?

Educational level. Find out the age upon leaving school/college and attainments if relevant.

Puberty/menstruation. Male:

How old were you when you first became aware of having erections? When did you first ejaculate? Did you have any problems related to going through puberty?

Female:

How old were you when you had your first period? Had you been warned in advance about this? Did you have any problems with your periods? How about now?

Work history.

Have you been in regular employment? What type? How about now? Do you find your work very demanding or tiring? What hours do you work? Do you have any stresses or worries related to your job? How secure is your current position?

Leisure and social activities (current and historical).

Do you have any hobbies, interests or activities? Do you go out much socially? Who with? What type of social events?

Do you have many friends? How much contact do you have with them? Did you make friends easily as a child?

Previous relationships.

How old were you when you first started dating? How serious were these relationships, how long did they last? How did you feel when they ended?

Have you been married before? Can you tell me about that?

Children and pregnancies.

Do you have any children? How old are they? Are they currently living with you? How do you get on as a family? Are there any problems related to the children that concern you?

Female:

Have you experienced any difficulties related to pregnancy? Have you suffered any miscarriages?

Non-sexual stress events.

Have you experienced any events in your life that caused you upset or worry? How about any illnesses or financial problems? Have there been any deaths in the family? When did this happen? How did it affect you? Have you ever experienced any psychiatric problems? (*Explore details.*)

Health items.

Are you currently taking any medication? What type is this? What is this for? How about in the past, have you had any major illnesses?

When did you last have a medical check-up? Do you find that you feel particularly tired and that this may interfere with your sex life?

Females:

Do you currently have any problems with your periods? If so, does this affect your sex life at all? (*For middle-aged females, the assessor should explore details regarding menopause and whether problems have been experienced.*)

Have you taken any non-prescription drugs such as LSD, heroin or amphetamines? How about previously?

How much alcohol do you drink each week? Do you drink most days?

See the earlier section concerning drug, alcohol and illness issues, plus the initial interview questions in Chapter 9.

Sexual history

It is important to explore the clients' previous sexual experiences and sexual development in order to identify the exact nature of the problem and any factors that may account for the current difficulties. Further information may be revealed regarding where and when the sexual dysfunction occurs or does not occur. Depending on the couple, the interviewer must decide whether to cover this section with the partners, either together or separately. Some clients may feel very reluctant to discuss sexual details in front of their partner, and it is advisable to ask each member of the partnership which format they would prefer. The following areas should be considered when taking a sexual history.

Early sexual experiences.

Can you remember playing sexual games as a child? How about as an adolescent? Can you recall any sexual foreplay or petting before you first had intercourse with someone? Did you find this arousing? What happened? Did you have an orgasm? Can you tell me about the first time you experienced orgasm and about the first time you had intercourse?

Do you know much about sex and how best to stimulate your partner? What books have you read about sex?

It is important for the assessor to confirm the accuracy of sexual knowledge at a later stage to ensure that the information held by the client with regard to anatomy and sexual techniques is correct.

Masturbation and self-pleasuring.

How old were you when you first started to masturbate? How often do you do this currently? How about in the past? Do you need any particular type of stimulation for orgasm when you masturbate? How would you describe your attitude towards masturbation?

Nocturnal penile tumescence and emissions (males).

Do you wake up either in the night or in the morning with an erect penis? If you haven't noticed, has your partner ever commented on this? Have you ever actually ejaculated in your sleep or during a dream? When was this . . . how often . . . does this still happen now?

Use of erotic materials and fantasy.

Do you get turned on by any particular things, like sexy pictures, stories or films? Which do you find most arousing? Are there any other things, like perfumes or music? Anything else? Do you or your partner use any of these things now to turn you on during sex? How about previously? Do you use any kinds of fantasies or imagination during sex? Can you tell me about these? How about when you masturbate?

Adult sexual relations.

Can you tell me about your sexual experiences as an adult? Have you been involved in sexual relationships before this one?

Did you become aroused during previous sexual relationships? Did you orgasm during these?

Previous sexual problems and treatments.

Have you experienced any sexual problems in any of your previous sexual relationships? Can you describe these? How long ago was this? Did you seek any treatment? Can you recall what action the therapist suggested? How successful was this? Have you had any other sexual difficulties in your current relationship?

Sexual stress events.

Have you experienced any events in your life that caused distress or worry that were related to sex or pregnancy?

It is important to consider events such as being raped, an incestuous relationship, an unwanted pregnancy or abortion. Bear in mind that the client may be reluctant to divulge this information initially, and it may be several sessions before sufficient trust is established to enable the client to disclose details relevant to such sensitive incidents.

Current relationship.

Nature of current relationship. Details of the current relationship need collecting from both a sexual and non-sexual perspective, as both may influence each partner's responsiveness during sex. Much information can be obtained from interview, but self-report inventories, as outlined later in this chapter, may provide a useful adjunct.

Can you tell me about the relationship you are involved in now? Are you married?

If not, ask about the frequency of contact, type of relationship, etc.

How long have you been together? How long did you go out together before you got married? Did you go away on a honeymoon? How did you get on sexually in the early stages of your relationship?

What attracted you to each other sexually in these early days?

Sexual experiences early in the relationship.

When did you first have sex together? Did you both orgasm when you first started having sex together? What kind of things have changed in your sexual relationship from then to now?

Common activities and interests.

What kinds of things do you do together besides sex? Do you spend much time chatting together? How often do you go out together as a couple? Would you like to spend more time together? Do you have many interests in common? What do you do together on a typical weekend?

Feelings of physical attraction, arousal and emotion.

Do you find your partner physically attractive? Does it turn you on to see him/her in the nude? Do you feel aroused when he/she touches you sexually? How would you best describe your feelings for your partner? Does this change during sex and if so, can you describe these feelings? Do you really want to have a good sexual relationship with your partner? How much do you want to have sex with him/her?

General satisfaction with the relationship.

How satisfactory is your relationship generally? Do you get on well together? Are there any aspects of your relationship, other than sex, that you would like to change? Does your partner have any habits that you feel are contributing to the difficulties the two of you are having sexually?

Communication between the couple.

How well do you communicate with each other? Do either of you find it hard to express your feelings? How about during sex, do you talk much then? Can you both say what things you would like the other to do? Do you actually ask? Do you say when you like something? What kinds of things would you say? How do you go about refusing sex when you don't feel like it? How about when you do feel like it, do you let your partner know?

Issues regarding contraception.

Are you or your partner using any form of contraception? *If so* . . . what type? Have you had any problems with this form of contraception? Do you have any worries about contraception? Do either of you have any worries about becoming pregnant?

Attitude regarding sex roles, self and treatment

Various aspects of the clients' cognitions can be explored at this stage. These may have important implications for maintenance of the problem and may need to be modified where maladaptive.

Ideals about sex.

How do you think a man should ideally behave sexually? How about a woman? How do you think you differ from this ideal? How about your partner? Can you describe to me how you would really like your sexual relationship to be? What kinds of activities would both do and how often?

Self-image.

Do you think your partner finds you sexually attractive? Do you feel attractive to the opposite sex? Do you feel that you are sufficiently masculine/feminine?

Sexual attitudes generally.

How would you describe your attitude to nudity . . . to masturbation . . . to sexual cleanliness? What are your feelings about sex during menstruation? Is this a problem at all in your sexual relationship? Do either of you find semen unpleasant? What about female lubrication, and its taste and smell?

Additional assessment considerations

Although it may seem that the content for the interview is enormously detailed, this is necessary given the great complexity of the human sexual response. The collection of data during assessment will generally involve two to three sessions prior to the onset of therapy. In addition to interview data, valuable information may also be obtained from a wide range of self-report instruments. These have the advantage of being less embarrassing to some clients and may be completed at home, saving professional time.

Specific assessment measures

Several instruments are available from which the clients' sexual behaviour and responsiveness can be assessed. The most well known of these is probably the 'sexual interaction inventory' (LoPiccolo & Steger, 1974), which has acceptable reliability and validity and has been shown to discriminate between sexually dysfunctional and non-dysfunctional couples. Other useful methods have been produced by Foster (1977) and Derogatis, Meyer & Dupkin (1976).

Sexual activities, experience and knowledge

The most widely used questionnaire in the area of sexual activity is the 'Bentler scale' (Bentler, 1967, 1968), which involves a list of 21 items relating to heterosexual behaviour and forms a cumulative, ordinal scale. Separate forms are available for males and females, and its psychometric properties are acceptable. The 'heterosexual behaviour inventory' (Robinson & Annon, 1975) is also useful, but details regarding reliability and validity are lacking. Finally, the 'sexual knowledge and attitude test' (Lief & Reed, 1972) is helpful in assessing a wider range of sexual activities and explores the client's attitudes and knowledge in relation to various aspects of sex. This measure has been widely researched and standardised, albeit with a student population.

Sexual arousal

The 'sexual arousal inventory' (Hoon, Hoon & Wincze, 1976) is a useful means of assessing arousal in women. This involves a list of 28 sexual activities that clients must rate on a 7-point Likert scale the degree to which arousal is affected adversely or positively. Its psychometric properties have been investigated with a population of North American women. A similar scale is available for men (Annon, 1975), but data regarding reliability, validity and norms are lacking.

Sexual anxiety

There is a lack of well-researched instruments for assessing sexual anxiety, but it is feasible to use methods such as the modified Bentler scale to ask clients to rate how much anxiety they experience with regard to specific sexual activities and situations. This approach has been used to assess sexual anxiety in treatment-outcome studies such as Spence (1985).

Having collected additional self-report questionnaire data, the assessor may also request that the clients complete various self-monitoring tasks. Direct observation of clients' sexual behaviour is not normally ethical or practical, hence it is necessary to rely on client observations from the natural setting. Many researchers emphasise the need for psychophysiological recordings to supplement assessment. Although this may provide valuable information, the necessary equipment is not available to the majority of therapists and is therefore not a focus of the present chapter.

Marital questionnaires

Various self-report measures exist for the assessment of marital satisfaction. The 'Locke-Wallace (1959) marital adjustment scale' was widely used for many years but is now frequently replaced by the 'Spanier (1976) dyadic adjustment scale'. This 32-item scale incorporates the 15 items of the Locke-Wallace scale, and has been factor-analysed to yield scales of consensus, satisfaction, cohesion and affectional expression. Alternatively, a total score may be used. The scale has been shown to discriminate well between distressed and non-distressed couples and has good psychometric properties (Spanier, 1976). Several other methods for the assessment of marital problems are available and the reader is referred to Margolin and Jacobson (1981) for a summary of these.

Treatment

Having identified the major determinants that are currently maintaining the clients' sexual problem, the assessor is in a position to design an individually tailored program suited to the needs of the client. A wide range of sex-therapy texts are available such as Masters & Johnson (1970), Jehu (1979), Kaplan (1974), and LoPiccolo & LoPiccolo (1978). Although such texts provide a valuable guide to therapy techniques, it is important that intervention does not become a package technique in which all clients with sexual dysfunctions within the same diagnostic label receive identical treatment components. The behavioural analysis produced by the assessment strategy outlined here should provide an important guide to the therapy components required for a particular couple or individual. The degree to which factors such as inadequate sexual knowledge, sexual anxiety, or maladaptive attitudes are important, will vary for different clients. Therapy should be tailored to meet the clients' needs, depending on the outcome of assessment.

Most behavioural approaches to the treatment of sexual dysfunction acknowledge the role played by a wide range of psychosocial variables in the determination of sexual problems. Hence, they aim to tackle the many educational aspects, anxiety components and attitudinal factors involved. Obviously, the exact content of the treatment programme varies according to the nature of the sexual dysfunction with which the clients present.

LoPiccolo and Stock (1986) provide an interesting review of the literature concerning the effectiveness of sex-therapy programmes. These authors conclude that results are particularly good for primary female orgasmic dysfunction and premature ejaculation. Secondary female orgasmic dysfunction is concluded to be more difficult to treat, as is erectile failure. LoPiccolo and Stock point out, however, the poor research methodology of many of the studies reviewed. Interestingly, a recent prospective study by Hawton, Catalan, Martin & Fagg (1986), reporting the long-term outcome of sex therapy, brings the above conclusions into question. Hawton *et al.* (1986) report poor results for premature ejaculation and yet good outcome for erectile dysfunction at 1–6 year follow-up. Long-term outcome for vaginismus was reported to be excellent, whereas female impaired sexual interest showed minimal improvement. Further studies of this type are needed before firm conclusions can be drawn about the long-term effectiveness of behavioural treatments of various types of sexual dysfunction.

7
Insomnia

Introduction

Insomnia may be defined as 'a chronic inability to obtain adequate sleep due to retarded sleep onset, frequent arousals, and/or early morning awakening' (Bootzin & Nicassio, 1978). Three principal categories of insomnia are implied in the above definition:

1. Difficulty falling asleep initially (sleep-onset insomnia; initial insomnia; early insomnia; predormital insomnia).
2. Interrupted sleep/frequent awakenings during the night (middle insomnia; restless sleep).
3. Awakening early in the morning with an inability to return to sleep (late insomnia; terminal insomnia).

The two latter categories are often referred to collectively as sleep-maintenance insomnia. The above classification is best considered as representing different types of insomnia, not types of individuals, since many insomniacs suffer from more than one of the above problems at various times. In addition, insomnia may be regarded as either primary or secondary in relation to aetiological considerations. Primary insomnia refers to the occurrence of sleep difficulties in the absence of other disorders, whereas the term 'secondary' insomnia refers to insomnia that may result from physical causes (e.g. pain, neurological damage) or other psychological problems (e.g. depression, manic-depressive disorders, alcohol abuse, etc.).

The Association of Sleep Disorders Centers has published guidelines for the diagnostic classification of sleep and arousal disorders (Association of Sleep Disorders, 1979; an abbreviated version is also available in the appendix of DSM-III, American Psychiatric Association, 1980). This classification scheme describes nine types of sleep disorders:

1. Psychophysiological insomnia.
2. Insomnia associated with psychiatric disorders.
3. Insomnia associated with use of drugs/alcohol.
4. Insomnia associated with respiratory impairment.
5. Insomnia associated with myoclonus/restless legs.
6. Insomnia associated with medical, toxic, environmental conditions.
7. Childhood-onset insomnia.
8. Insomnia associated with polysomnographic disturbances.
9. No objective abnormality, but reports of 'subjective' insomnia.

However, the scheme for the classification of insomnia has been replaced in DSM-III-R (APA, 1987) by categories of: (1) primary insomnia (not associated with any other mental or organic disorder); (2) insomnia related to another mental disorder, such as major depression or anxiety disorder; and (3) insomnia related to a known organic factor such as sleep apnoea, arthritis, substance-abuse disorder or use of medication.

Intermittent insomnia is reported by 21–35 per cent of the population, the variation in figures being due to differences in the survey method employed in the various studies. The incidence of chronic, severe insomnia is obviously lower, probably in the order of 10–13 per cent (Mellinger, Balter & Uhlenhuth, 1985). Although insomnia is more common in psychiatric populations, it may also occur in individuals with no other apparent psychological disturbance.

A question that frequently arises in relation to the definition of insomnia is: how much sleep is it necessary or sufficient for an individual to receive? This question is more complex than it may at first appear. A sleep-onset latency of more than 30 minutes or a total sleep time of less than 6.5 hours are conventional criteria for insomnia in research studies. The average sleep-onset latency of non-insomniacs is about 20–23 minutes, with an average of 35 minutes being spent awake after initial sleep onset (Kales & Kales, 1984). Total sleep time decreases as age increases, mainly due to a higher frequency and longer duration of awakenings during the night, while sleep-onset latency is not markedly affected by age (Kales & Kales, 1984). DSM-III-R requires that the insomnia has occurred:

> at least three times for at least one month and is sufficiently severe to result in either a complaint of significant daytime fatigue or the observation by others of some symptom that is attributable to the sleep disturbance, e.g., irritability or impaired daytime functioning (p. 300).

In assessing total sleep time, the clinician needs to take into account any daytime naps that may tend to reduce the need for prolonged night-time sleep, especially in the elderly. It should also be kept in mind that individuals vary in the amount of sleep that they require in order to function effectively during the day, and that this subjective factor needs to be considered in the clinical assessment of the individual.

Physiology of sleep

At this point, it might be useful to take a digression into some general matters concerning the physiology of sleep. The sleep cycle is classified into four stages, plus rapid eye movement (REM) sleep, based on electroencephalographic (EEG), electro-oculographic (EOG) and electromyographic (EMG) patterns. Stage 1 refers to the transition from wakefulness to sleep, and may recur after body movements during sleep. Stage 2 consists of a relatively low-amplitude, mixed-frequency EEG pattern with little eye movement and reduced EMG levels. Stages 3 and 4 are referred to as slow-wave sleep since they consist of a high-amplitude, low-frequency EEG pattern. REM sleep involves bursts of rapid eye movements and a low-amplitude/mixed-frequency EEG pattern. EMG levels are at their lowest during this stage, but other indices of activity are heightened (e.g. penile erections, increased oxygen consumption, increased body temperature). Normal sleep involves a progression from Stage 1 through to Stage 4, then a return to Stages 3 and 2, followed by REM sleep. This cycle, which takes about 90 minutes to complete, is repeated approximately four to six times per night, with increases in the amount of time spent in REM sleep and decreases in the duration of Stages 3 and 4 as the cycle is repeated. It appears that a small percentage of insomniacs may have atypical polysomnographic features (such as repeated REMs during non-REM sleep), but it is not possible to conclude from the existing evidence that insomniacs as a group differ from non-insomniacs in any systematic way on the various polysomnographic features of sleep.

Insomnia and medical conditions

The clinician needs to be aware that insomnia may occur in conjunction with a number of medical conditions, e.g. cardiovascular disease, respiratory disorders, gastrointestinal disorders and chronic renal insufficiency. In some cases, insomnia may be a result of the psychological impact of the knowledge that one has a major disorder, or due to fears of having a life-threatening episode during the night. Sleep apnoea, nocturnal myoclonus, chronic pain, headache, or tinnitus (ringing in the ears) may contribute to insomnia. Sleep apnoea refers to abnormal respiratory irregularity during sleep, involving periods in which breathing may cease for about 10 seconds. The person may experience a choking sensation, and the episode is often associated with snorting and gasping sounds. Nocturnal myoclonus refers to periodic jerking of the legs during sleep. Both these conditions may result in the person waking up, although cases of insomnia connected with apnoea or myoclonus are relatively rare.

Ingestion of substances

A number of medicines and foods may contribute to insomnia, e.g. stimulants, benzodiazepines, hypnotics, non-prescription drugs, caffeine and alcohol. Questions about the ingestion of these substances and about general diet should be included in the initial interview. Some individuals seem to be particularly sensitive to caffeine (contained in coffee, tea and cola drinks). Cigarette-smoking may also aggravate sleep difficulties. Prolonged use of hypnotics and benzodiazepines, often prescribed for the treatment of insomnia, may actually disrupt normal sleep, and reduce the amount of REM sleep, although occasional use of such medicines may be therapeutically useful.

Coexisting psychological conditions

Insomnia may be the principal or sole complaint in many individuals who seek treatment. Tan, Kales, Kales, Soldatos and Bixler (1984) report that DSM-III diagnoses of dysthymic, anxiety, somatoform and substance-abuse disorders were very common amongst insomniacs. The clinician should be particularly careful to check for features of depression, and may find it useful to consult Chapter 3 (this volume) for details of the assessment of depressive disorders. Early-morning wakening or sleep-onset insomnia occur in about one-third of depressed individuals. Anxiety and tension are also very commonly reported by insomniacs. Thus, the clinician should thoroughly check the presence of cognitive, physiological and behavioural features of anxiety during the period leading up to bedtime, when actually in bed and during the day. The reader should also consult Chapter 2 of this text for further details on the assessment of anxiety.

Theories of insomnia

Two principal theories have emerged concerning the role of psychological factors in the aetiology of insomnia, one of which involves the suggestion that there is an elevation of physiological arousal at or near bedtime, the others concerning the role of stimulus-control over the onset of sleep.

The hyperarousal theory suggests that insomniacs experience an increase in heart rate, muscle tension and other physiological indices of arousal at, or near, bedtime, producing a state that is incompatible with the physiological conditions required for sleep onset. Consistent with this theory, several researchers have demonstrated that insomniacs experience higher heart rates and/or EMG levels prior to sleep (e.g. Freedman & Sattler, 1982; Haynes, Adams & Franzen, 1981; Monroe, 1967), although such EMG elevations were not obtained by Frankel, Coursey, Buchbinder & Snyder (1976) or Freedman & Papsdorf (1976). However, it should be noted that large individual differences in resting heart rate and EMG are obtained in most investigations, and that the correlation between physiological arousal and sleep-onset time is very low. In addition, the factors that are responsible for hyperarousal at bedtime have not been clearly elucidated. One might conjecture that a high level of stress during the day, ruminations about past or future events or worrying about the consequences of a sleepless night may all be likely to lead to heightened arousal in susceptible individuals.

The relationship between stressful life events and insomnia has been the subject of surprisingly little research. Healey, Kales, Monroe, Bixler, Chamberlain and Soldatos (1981) report that, relative to a control group consisting of good sleepers, insomniacs had higher scores on a measure of the occurrence of life-events coinciding with the year in which their insomnia had its onset. Most of the events reported were undesirable events, many of which involved a loss of some kind, or an exit from the social field. Since these kinds of events are typical of those associated with the onset of depression (e.g. Paykel *et al.*, 1969), it is quite likely that the onset of insomnia was connected with a depressive syndrome in a large proportion of the sample. While there is clearly a need for further research in this area, the research of Healey *et al.* suggests that the clinician should examine carefully the period surrounding the onset of the insomnia in order to explore the role of environmental factors in the aetiology of the person's current problems. It should be noted that insomnia may commence due to a set of circumstances that are no longer in operation, although the insomnia has continued. For example, insomnia that has developed as a side effect of drugs or during a stay in hospital may have continued in spite of the cessation of the triggering factors. It is possible that, once initiated, other factors such as the expectation of sleep difficulties or a conditioned elevation of arousal may serve to maintain the insomnia.

The other major approach to the aetiology of insomnia is represented by the stimulus-control theory (Bootzin & Nicassio, 1978). A central tenet of this theory is the assertion that the onset of sleep in normal sleepers is assisted by the pairing of stimuli in the bedroom with sleep. It is suggested that insomnia may develop due to the failure of relevant cues in the bed and bedroom to act as discriminative stimuli for sleep. The person may engage in sleep-incompatible behaviours such as reading, watching TV, or eating in the bed or bedroom, thus reducing the strength of the stimuli in the bed or bedroom to promote conditions necessary for sleep. Bootzin and Nicassio (1978) describe a treatment programme based on this theory, in which the person is instructed to (1) go to bed only when sleepy; (2) lie in bed awake for no longer than 10 minutes; (3) get up after this time and go to another room; (4) return to bed only when sleepy; (5) not take naps during the day;

and (6) rise at the same time each morning. Although the evidence for the efficacy of this treatment is now quite substantial (e.g. Lacks, Bertelson, Gans & Kinkel, 1983; Turner & Ascher, 1979), it appears that neither all the components are necessary, nor that the procedure achieves its effects for reasons postulated by the theory (e.g. Zwart & Lisman, 1979). There has been relatively little study of the hypothesis that insomniacs engage in a greater amount of sleep-incompatible behaviours in the bed or bedroom in comparison to non-insomniacs. Haynes, Follingsted & McGowan (1974) found no difference between insomniacs and normal sleepers in the number of sleep-incompatible behaviours, although the measure consisted only of two retrospective, self-report questionnaire items. In a later set of studies, in which a variety of methodologies were employed, Haynes, Adams, West, Kamens & Safranek (1982) failed to find any evidence in support of the stimulus-control hypothesis. Some support is offered by a study of Kazarian, Howe & Csapo (1979) who developed a questionnaire designed to assess the extent of engagement in sleep-incompatible behaviours. It was found that insomniacs obtained a higher mean score on this questionnaire than a non-insomniac control group, and that a subset of the items discriminated insomniacs from non-insomniacs.

It should be noted that psychological theorists have mainly focused on the aetiology of sleep-onset insomnia, and have generally paid little attention to middle or late insomnia. As mentioned earlier in this chapter, the sleep laboratory research indicates that even normal sleepers are awake for brief periods during the night as part of the regular sleep cycle. Thus, it could be argued that the wakening in insomniacs is part of any normal sleep pattern, and is not in need of specific explanation. Once awake, however, some insomniacs have difficulty returning to sleep, and this aspect of the problem needs to be addressed by any general psychological theory of insomnia. According to the hyperarousal theory, it would be suggested that such individuals may already be more aroused even during sleep, or that they may easily become aroused once they are awake, particularly if they begin to engage in cognitive activity (e.g. thinking about past or future events, or worrying about the consequences of a sleepless night, etc.).

The role of cognitions in insomnia, which has been mentioned in passing in this chapter, has also been the subject of a small amount of research. It may be argued that cognitive activity plays an important role in the onset or maintenance of insomnia, either through an effect on arousal or through some more direct means, although evidence to support this view is rather scant, and in some cases, contradictory. For example, Freedman & Sattler (1982) found no differences between insomniacs and non-insomniacs on a measure of pre-sleep cognitive activity. Lichstein & Rosenthal (1980) found that a large majority of sleep-onset insomniacs subjectively report cognitive arousal or a combination of cognitive and physical arousal prior to sleep. Of course, it is possible that such cognitive activity, if it does occur, is simply an epiphenomenon of sleep disturbance: a result of the activity of the mind in an already aroused state. Nevertheless, there are some individuals for whom cognitive activity may be sufficiently distressing that it ought to form a focus of attention in a comprehensive treatment programme. Nicassio, Mendlowitz, Fussell & Petras (1985) suggest that pre-sleep arousal may be divisible into somatic and cognitive components, and that individuals may vary with respect to the involvement of each of these components in their sleep disturbance. Nicassio *et al.* (1985) have developed the 'pre-sleep arousal scale', a measure that has been designed to assess both the cognitive and somatic levels of pre-sleep arousal. This scale might be employed for the purpose of identifying individuals for whom one or other of these hypothesised types of arousal is most problematic.

Specific assessment methods

A number of techniques may be useful in the assessment of insomnia, such as daily sleep diaries, polysomnography, electronic sleep-monitoring devices and partner observations.

Daily sleep diaries

A sleep diary consists of a set of forms on which the client is asked to record various aspects of his or her sleep each morning. Such devices provide a useful means of obtaining baseline data concerning the initial severity of the problem and for monitoring response to treatment. The questions involve (1) estimates of sleep parameters such as sleep-onset latency, frequency of awakenings during the night and total time spent asleep; and (2) ratings of qualitative aspects such as tension, mood and restlessness. An

Table 7.1: *Daily sleep diary*

Day...Date...

Last night: How long did it take for you to fall asleep? ....

How many times did you wake up during the night? ....

How long were you awake at each wakening? (1)........(2)........(3)........(4)........

How much sleep did you have in total?...

Did you take any medication? If so, please give details...................................

How would you describe your mood this morning?

Circle one: Very good   Good   Fair   Low   Very low

Can you recall what you were thinking about last night as you tried to fall asleep?

....

....

How tense or uptight were you feeling last night while you were trying to fall asleep?

Circle one: Very tense   Moderately tense   A little tense   Not tense   Relaxed

example of this kind of form is contained in Table 7.1. Such devices have been demonstrated to possess good test-retest reliability, and have been found to correlate highly with other forms of assessment (Bootzin & Engle-Friedman, 1981). However, it appears that insomniacs overestimate their sleep-onset latencies in comparison with EEG and objectively-determined sleep onset, and that they tend to underestimate the number of awakenings during the night (Lovibond, 1979).

Polysomnography

This term refers to the measurement of physiological parameters such as EEG, EMG and EOG during the course of sleep. Clients usually sleep in a specially equipped laboratory for three or more nights. The first night is regarded as an adaptation night, providing the individual with an opportunity to adjust to the novel equipment and surroundings. EEG tracings can be used to measure sleep-onset latency, nocturnal awakenings and the amount of time spent in each stage of sleep. Such data may reveal departures from self-reported latencies and awakenings, and may indicate unusual sleep patterns, sleep apnoea and other abnormalities. EMG tracings may also be useful to indicate periods of heightened arousal prior to or during sleep, helping to clarify the relationship between hyperarousal and insomnia in the individual case. Obviously, polysomnography is a very time-consuming, expensive and inconvenient procedure, and it suggested that such detailed investigations be reserved for clients who (1) show particularly poor response to the initial stages of treatment; (2) report unusual features of sleep disturbance or additional problems such as nocturnal headaches; (3) are unable to provide clear information about the nature of their sleep problem; or (4) display evidence of sleep apnoea or nocturnal myoclonus. Devices are now available that enable polysomnography to be performed in the client's home, with the transmission of data to the clinic or laboratory being achieved via the telephone cable (e.g., Rosekind, Coates & Thoresen, 1978). Such equipment has the advantage of providing measurement in the person's natural sleeping environment over longer periods of time than would be possible with the laboratory-based method, although the person (or partner) needs to be carefully trained in the electrode-placement procedure.

Electronic monitoring devices

An objective measure of insomnia, the sleep monitor, has been developed by Lovibond (1979; see also Birrell, 1983). This apparatus consists of a button that is either placed in the bed or is taped to the person's hand and a recording instrument located at the bedside. The instrument emits a very faint tone at regular preset intervals (e.g. every 10 minutes) to which the person responds, if awake, by pressing the button. The button presses are recorded for later analysis, allowing the calculation of the estimated sleep-onset latency, time awake during the night and total sleep time. Most individuals are reported to adapt to the use of the device within a couple of nights (Young, 1982). Comparisons with EEG-determined sleep have been conducted that provide good support for the validity and reliability of this device (Birrell, 1983). Kelley & Lichstein (1980) have developed a similar device that emits a tone every 10 minutes to which the person responds with a verbal acknowledgement that is recorded on audiotape. This apparatus has also been shown to result in a high degree of concordance with EEG sleep criteria (Lichstein, Nickel, Hoelscher & Kelley, 1982). Devices such as these have a distinct advantage over self-report assessments both in permitting all-night recording of several sleep parameters, and in reducing the effects of memory artefacts, demand characteristics and various sources of error.

Partner observations

Certain researchers have employed observations made by a sleeping partner or significant other as an adjunct to self-report data (Tokarz & Lawrence, 1974). The partner is provided with a set of specific criteria by which they are to determine whether or not the person is asleep. The criteria suggested by Tokarz and Lawrence are as follows:

1. Eyes closed.
2. No voluntary movements for at least 10 minutes.
3. Rate of respiration less than normal.
4. No response to the question, 'are you asleep?'.

Sleep-onset latencies estimated by this method have been found to be highly correlated with self-ratings ($r = .91$ to $.99$). There are clearly some practical problems that limit the usefulness of the procedure, such as the difficulty for the non-insomniac partner in staying awake long enough to observe the insomniac's sleep latency! The use of this procedure may be best reserved for those cases in which one seriously suspects the validity of the self-ratings or where self-rating presents particular difficulties for the client.

Behavioural aspects

There are several behavioural aspects of insomnia that may be assessed apart from the conventional sleep parameters. The stimulus-control theory would suggest that the clinician should assess the amount of time spent engaging in sleep-incompatible behaviours in the bed or bedroom. The 'sleep behaviour ratings scale' developed by Kazarian *et al.* (1979) would be useful for this task. Measures of daily stress, as discussed in the chapter on headaches, may also be useful. These questionnaires include: the 'unpleasant events schedule' (UES; Lewinsohn, Marmelstein, Alexander & MacPhillamy, 1985) and the 'hassles scale' (Kanner, Coyne, Schaefer & Lazarus, 1981). A scale designed to measure the amount and kind of cognitive activity related to insomnia has also been developed recently (Wilson & Forbes, 1987).

The interview

The purpose of the interview should be to obtain information about the features of the person's insomniac problem and to identify likely aetiological factors. Such information ought to lead to a rational basis for the choice of treatment intervention. Information on the sleep-onset latency, number of awakenings and so forth should be backed up by some more detailed measurement as described above. The following is a guide to the kinds of questions that the person who complains of insomnia could be asked in the course of an interview.

General features

What kind of difficulty do you have with your sleep — is it a problem for you to get off to sleep at night, or do you find yourself waking up earlier than you would like?
How long does it generally take for you to get to sleep?
How many nights each week would you say are like that?
How long did you take to get to sleep last night? Is that a typical night for you lately?
Do you wake up often during the night? How often? How long do you stay awake for? About what time(s) do you wake up?
How about last night — did you wake up during the night? (*Obtain more details.*)
What time do you usually wake up in the morning? (*Find out details about the range of wakening times, etc.*)
Do you use an alarm?
What time did you wake up this morning?

By this point you will have ascertained which of the principal types of insomnia (early, middle or late) is of most concern to the person. You might then try to obtain more details relevant to the type that is most problematic for the person. Here, we will proceed with questions related to each type in turn.

Bedtime

What time do you usually go to bed? (*Check range.*)

How long is this after you have had dinner?

What kinds of things do you generally do in the evening?

Go over the events of a typical evening, e.g. you could check on the previous few evenings.

What sort of things do you eat or drink between dinner and going to bed?

Check specifically on coffee, tea, alcohol or other drugs.

When you go to bed, do you spend any time in bed reading, watching TV, listening to the radio, etc.

How tired do you feel when you go bed?

What happens if you discover that you are having difficulty getting to sleep? What do you do?

Do you get up after a while, or turn on the light?

What do you do if you get up?

Do you like doing these things at that time?

How long would you usually stay up before going back to bed?

If you are lying in bed, trying to get to sleep, how do you feel? Sometimes people notice that they are tensed up, you know, muscles feeling tight, or a clenched jaw, or your heart beating fast. Do you ever notice these sorts of feelings when you are trying to get to sleep?

Do you notice any other sorts of feelings?

Cognitive activity

These questions are designed to lead into discussion about the thoughts in which the person engages when lying in bed awake. It would be important to follow up many of these questions with more detailed investigation of the sources of worry, or problems with which they may be attempting to cope.

What sort of things do you think about while you are trying to get to sleep?

You might need to make some suggestions here, for example:

Do you worry about what you'll be like the next day if you can't get to sleep? How often?

Do you get annoyed that you can't sleep? How often?

Do you find yourself going over events of the day?

What sorts of events do you think about? How often?

Do you find yourself thinking about tomorrow, making plans, etc. What kinds of plans? How often?

How do you feel while you are thinking about these sorts of things?

Are there any particular things that you keep thinking about?

(*Here, you might look for topics such as financial worries, interpersonal concerns, work problems, etc.*)
To what extent are you able to control such thoughts if you try?

Morning

What time do you usually get up in the morning? (*range*)
How do you feel in the morning when you wake up?

Stimulus-control

Here, one is looking for evidence of poor stimulus-control. It is a good idea to ask about specific activities such as reading, studying, watching TV, talking on the telephone, etc.

Do you ever take a nap during the day? How often? How long?
How much time do you spend in the bedroom, doing things other than sleeping or napping, during the day? What sorts of the things do you do?
Do you watch TV in the bedroom or listen to the radio?
Do you study/work in the bedroom?
How well do you sleep when you stay somewhere other than your home, e.g. when you are on holiday, or staying at someone's house, etc?

Correlations with daily events

Do you notice any differences in your ease of getting to sleep, depending on what day of the week it is? Is any one day particularly bad? Is it easier at weekends?
Do you notice any differences in your ease of getting to sleep depending on what you have done during the day? (*Explore details.*)
How do you spend a typical day?

It is important to try to gauge the person's level of activity, exercise, the amount of time spent in stressful tasks, the amount of time spent in relaxing and engaging in enjoyable activities, etc.

How much tea or coffee do you consume during the day?
What about other drinks such as alcohol?
Do you notice whether the insomnia is affected by any activities that are planned for the following day?

Consequences

In this section, you need to look for both the positive and negative consequences of the sleeping problem. Positive consequences may include the ability to disengage oneself from certain activities.

To what extent does your sleeping difficulty affect the things you do?
Do you complain to others of feeling tired?
Does this mean that you sometimes don't do certain things because of your tiredness? (*Find out details.*)
How does your sleeping difficulty affect other members of your family (*or significant others if relevant*)?
How does your spouse/partner react to your sleeping problem?
Does he/she complain that it is disrupting his/her sleep?
Does it affect them in any other way?

Previous night

Another useful strategy is to investigate the previous night (or the most recent troublesome night) in some detail, by asking questions such as the following:

Let's now spend some time going over a recent difficult night, e.g. last night — how did you sleep last night?

If last night was a fairly good night, just work back over the recent period until a troublesome night is obtained.

What time did you go to bed?
How did you feel when you went to bed?
What time did you fall asleep?
Can you remember what you were thinking about while you were lying awake?

Explore this area in more detail:

Once you were asleep, did you wake up again during the night?
How many times?
What time of the night was it when you woke up?
How long did you stay awake for?
What did you do when you were awake?
Did you get up? *If 'yes'*, how long did you stay up?

In addition, it is important to obtain a general medical history, and to enquire into the treatments that have been tried previously and any current medication (see Chapter 1 for details). Sleep apnoea or other unusual disturbances, if suspected, should be further investigated in a sleep laboratory. It would also be necessary to evaluate the level of depression (see Chapter 3), anxiety (see Chapter 2) and other psychological difficulties that may be discerned or suspected during the interview.

Treatment of insomnia

Approaches to the treatment of insomnia have been derived from both the hyperarousal and the stimulus-control theories. The hyperarousal theory suggests that techniques such as relaxation training would be beneficial, and there is a good deal of research supporting the effectiveness of this approach with insomnia (see Borkovec, 1982 for a review of this area). Details of the stimulus-control treatment can be found in Bootzin & Nicassio (1978). There is also a growing literature on the use of a cognitive approach referred to as paradoxical intention, in which the person is instructed to try to stay awake (Ascher & Efran, 1978; Lacks *et al.*, 1983; Turner & Ascher, 1979). In general, each of these treatments has some supportive evidence for its effectiveness.

It is possible that individuals vary in their response to these different treatments, although little research has been directed at this issue. Hauri (1981) and Hauri, Percy, Hellekson, Hartmann & Russ (1982) found that anxious and tense patients responded best to relaxation training and that the less tense subjects responded best to an alternative treatment involving sensorimotor rhythm feedback. Shealey, Lowe & Ritzler (1980) reported that improvement in a combined relaxation-training/stimulus-control treatment was associated with scores on the MMPI subscales (high test-taking attitude, *D*, psychopathic deviate subscores and low *Hy*, hypomania, *Sc*, and *F* scores). There is a need for further studies on the value of differential prognostic indicators so that treatments may be better tailored to individual differences in the features or aetiology of insomnia. At this stage, it would seem profitable to conduct a careful assessment of the extent to which the person experiences symptoms of either depression or anxiety/tension, and the degree to which either stimulus-control problems, a high level of daily stress, or hyperarousal at bedtime contributes to the insomnia. A high level of depression would indicate the need for the therapist to consider the direct treatment of the depressive features using treatments that have been found to be effective for depressions (see Chapter 3). The presence of high levels of somatic or cognitive arousal might be used as an indication of the need for relaxation techniques (Bernstein & Borkovec, 1973) in the former or other more cognitive approaches in the latter (e.g. Mitchell, 1979; Mitchell & White, 1977). On the other hand, evidence of poor stimulus-control would indicate that the stimulus-control treatment might provide a useful starting point for therapy. The principal aim of the present chapter has been to draw attention to the need to assess the problem of insomnia on several dimensions and to select an appropriate intervention accordingly. It is suggested that treatments could be tailored to follow from the dimension of most relevance to the individual.

Further reading

For more detailed discussion of general aspects of sleep and insomnia, it is recommended that you read the book by Kales and Kales (1984). Borkovec (1982) provides a valuable summary of the theoretical and treatment-outcome literature. The recent manual by Lacks (1987) would be a helpful guide to therapeutic interventions.

8
Headaches

Introduction

Headache complaints constitute one of the most common areas of concern amongst patients who seek medical treatment. It has been estimated that about 40 per cent of the adult population experience regular headaches (Ziegler, Hassanein & Couch, 1977). During the past 15 years, psychologists have proposed various treatment approaches that appear to be effective with many headache sufferers. Such treatments include relaxation training, biofeedback, and, more recently, cognitive therapy. When the clinician interviews a person who presents with chronic headaches, it is necessary to obtain a detailed account of the features and history of the headache attacks, antecedent events and consequences and the cognitive, physiological and behavioural aspects of the problem. Information obtained from such assessment will assist in the selection of particular treatment components. The aim of the present chapter is to indicate how to conduct this type of interview with patients who present with headaches.

Features of headaches

One of the major issues in the assessment of headache patients concerns the classification of headaches. The Ad Hoc Committee on the Classification of Headache (1962) identified 15 different categories of headaches. Many of these categories included headaches related to opthalmological disorders, organic disorders, sinus, head injury and other medical problems. There are four classes of headaches in which psychological factors may be implicated: (1) migraine (or vascular) headache; (2) tension (or muscle-contraction) headache; (3) combined migraine and tension headache; and (4) headache of delusional, conversion or hypochondriachal states (sometimes referred to as psychogenic headache). A major controversy exists concerning the validity of this classification scheme, a point that will be discussed in more detail in a subsequent section.

The term 'migraine' is usually applied to headaches that are characterised by some of the following features:

1. Prodromal signs (visual and other sensory disturbances, e.g. flashing lights, numbness, tingling, or other sensations that generally occur prior to the headache).
2. Vomiting and/or nausea.
3. Unilateral headache, especially at the onset of the headache, although in some patients the pain may become bilateral as the headache develops.
4. Throbbing or pulsating ache.

Migraine headaches also tend to have a sudden onset, the pain is often very severe, and may be accompanied by photophobia (sensitivity to light) or sonophobia (sensitivity to sound).

Migraine sufferers are usually categorised as either (1) classic; (2) common; or (3) cluster types. *Classic migraine* is characterised by the presence of prodromal features — the pain is usually unilateral and nausea/vomiting frequently accompany the headache. The term *common migraine* is generally used to refer to predominately bilateral migraine headaches without the prodromal signs. *Cluster headaches* are so-named because of the unusual temporal pattern, typically occurring numerous times during a relatively short period of time (one to four weeks), after which there may be total remission of symptoms for several months or even years until the cycle is repeated.

Migraine headaches are thought to involve two phases of vascular aberration. The first phase consists of vasoconstriction of a portion of the cranial arteries. This vasoconstriction results in a reduced blood flow to the cranial area and decreased levels of oxygen in the affected areas. In response to such effects, vasodilation of cranial arteries is thought to be triggered via a mechanism that is responsible for maintaining adequate cranial blood flow. Such vasodilation leads to an increased blood flow, but also leads to distention of the cranial arteries, local inflammation and oedema. Pain may be experienced as blood is pumped through the affected areas. It is thought that the inflammatory reaction is aggravated by a biochemical process, possibly involving the release of histamines, neurokinin or other substances. There is also evidence that lowered levels of the neurotransmitter, serotinin (a vasoconstrictor of scalp arteries and a CNS pain inhibitor), may be associated with migraine attacks.

Tension headache represents the second major category. As the name suggests, these headaches are thought to be caused by excessive or prolonged contraction of the muscles of the neck, scalp, shoulders and face. The Ad Hoc Committee for the Classification of Headache (1962) defines tension headache as an 'ache or sensation of tightness, pressure or constriction, widely varied in intensity, frequency and duration, sometimes long lasting and commonly sub-occipital' (p. 717). Tension headaches usually involve a feeling of tightness or pressure, pain in the neck, a dull, continuous headache. They are often bilateral. In practice, tension headaches are often diagnosed more by exclusion criteria (i.e. the absence of typical migranous features) rather than by the presence of specific signs and symptoms. It is also widely considered that migraine and tension headaches differ in their frequency of occurrence — migraine attacks commonly occur from one to four times per month (Selby & Lance, 1960), whereas tension headaches tend to occur much more regularly, even daily or continuously.

The Ad Hoc Committee also defines a *combined* vascular and muscle-contraction headache as 'combinations of vascular headache of the migraine type and muscle-contraction headache prominently coexisting in an attack' (p. 718), although the terms 'combined' or 'mixed' headaches are sometimes employed to refer to patients who report these two patterns of headaches on different occasions.

The final type of headache defined by the Ad Hoc Committee in which psychological factors may operate is referred to as 'headache of delusional, conversion, or hypochondriacal states'. These are 'headaches of illnesses in which the prevailing clinical disorder is a delusional or a conversion reaction and a peripheral pain mechanism is nonexistent. Closely allied are the hypochondriacal reactions in which the peripheral disturbances relevant to headache are minimal' (Ad Hoc Committee, p. 718). This type of headache is very rarely discussed in the literature, possibly because the condition itself is not commonly found. The clinician ought to be alert to the existence of psychogenic headache, particularly in patients for whom there is independent evidence of hypochondriasis, hysteria, and conversion reactions. For further discussion of the features and nature of migraine headaches, the reader is referred to Adams, Feuerstein & Fowler (1980).

Problems in the classification of headache

The use of the terms 'migraine' and 'tension' headache implies the existence of two distinct types of headache. However, this dichotomous classification scheme has been seriously challenged by the research evidence. Migraine-headache sufferers have been found to have higher resting EMG levels than tension-headache patients (Philips, 1978; Pozniak-Patewicz, 1976), suggesting that heightened muscle tension may be implicated in migraine headaches to an even greater extent than in tension headaches. Many patients who are diagnosed as suffering from tension headache present with at least one of the typical migrainous symptoms, making any distinction between the two types rather more problematic than would appear from the listing of characteristics (Bakal & Kaganov, 1977). In fact, a very large proportion of headache patients are difficult to diagnose as migraine- or tension-headache types because of the mixture of features that are frequently present. Bakal (1982), one of the strongest critics of the dichotomous classification, has suggested that there may be a single fundamental psychobiological process that underlies both migraine and tension headaches, and that there may be a continuum of severity that manifests itself in the presence of a wider range of symptoms. Although many researchers appear to be sympathetic with this view, the diagnostic system based on the Ad Hoc Committee's (1962) recommendations has generally not been abandoned. Overall, there seems to be little recognition of the fact that there is a fundamental difficulty in deciding whether distinctions in symptomatology represent basic differences in aetiology or differences in the expression of a single aetiological process. While there could very well be a single causal factor that is expressed in different ways depending on physiological differences between individuals, it is still possible that such physiological differences may necessitate somewhat different treatment or preventative approaches. The problems concerning the existing system for the classification of headache are unlikely to be resolved until we know a great deal more about the psychological processes involved in headaches and the ways in which such processes interact. There also needs to be a much greater attention given to the possible differences that may exist between the various subtypes of migraine headaches (Ruff, Moss & Lombardo, 1986). The authors are in agreement with Thompson (1982) who argues that abandonment of the present classification system at this stage would be premature.

Theories of headaches

It is difficult to identify a specific behavioural theory of the aetiology of headache. However, most psychological treatments of headaches are based on the assumption that headache is a result of exposure to stress, which leads to prolonged or excessive contraction of the musculature, especially in the neck, scalp, shoulder and face. Relative to non-headache controls, higher EMG frontalis resting levels have been observed in headache sufferers in several studies (e.g. Andrasik & Holroyd, 1980; Martin & Mathews, 1978; Philips, 1977), although Bakal and Kaganov (1977) failed to support this finding. It is also possible that stress factors may lead to vascular changes, either through some biochemical mediation process, or as a result of muscle tension. Environmental stressors or 'triggers' could include interpersonal difficulties, work pressures and so forth. Of course, such triggers would be likely to be highly idiosyncratic. Furthermore, cognitive theorists argue that the individual's appraisal of events represents an important component in the link between environmental events and the occurrence of symptoms. Bakal (1982) rejects the idea that environmental stressors play a significant role in headaches other than for those people who only experience headaches irregularly, or early in the development of chronic headache. Instead, he suggests that a very important factor is the individual's reaction to the onset of a headache, or their expectation that they will have a headache in certain circumstances once a chronic pattern has been established.

Some researchers have suggested that there may be a particular 'headache personality', consisting of anxious, obsessive, perfectionistic traits. However, the research evidence is quite inconsistent with respect to this question, and much of the research is fraught with methodological inadequacies (Harrison, 1975).

Consistent with some of this literature, Kearney, Wilson & Haralambous (1987) found evidence of elevations in anxiety and depression in comparison to non-headache clinical and normal control groups. Close inspection of the data revealed that this mean difference was contributed by relatively few individual headache sufferers who demonstrated clinical levels of pathology. Thus, it would be reasonable to conclude that some, but not all, headache sufferers show a marked degree of anxious and depressive symptomatology. For reviews of the psychological and physiological factors involved in headaches, see Blanchard & Andrasik (1982) or Williamson (1981).

Background to interview

In the section that follows, suggestions are made about the areas of inquiry that are relevant to complete a thorough initial interview with a patient who suffers from headaches. Such an interview should result in detailed information concerning: (1) history of the headache problem; (2) specific physiological, behavioural and cognitive features of the headaches; and (3) possible causal or maintenance factors. Given the variety of possible causes of headaches, the questions are deliberately intended to cover a broad range of possible causal and diagnostic factors, although a cognitive-behavioural emphasis is evident. It is also important that the clinician be alert to the possibility that psychological factors may not necessarily play a role in the aetiology of the headache problem of a specific individual. *The need for independent medical investigation cannot be overemphasised.* Headache sufferers should always be referred to a general physician, or, in some cases, to specialists in the area of neurology, opthalmology, dentistry and other areas as the need arises.

Although referral for medical examination should be a routine part of the assessment of headaches, this practice ought to be followed especially if the headache problem has developed very recently, or there has been a recent physical injury or illness or a history of previous illnesses such as cancer or vascular disorders, or if the headache is accompanied by unusual features such as short stabbing aches, continuous pain or non-pain sensations. It is important to keep in mind that headache problems may be a symptom of serious medical disorders, e.g. brain tumor, for which psychological interventions would be entirely inappropriate.

Headaches may also occur in conjunction with temporomandibular joint dysfunction (TMJ) and other myofascial pain disorders (Ruff *et al.*, 1986; also see Moss, Garrett & Chiodo, 1982 for a general discussion of TMJ and orofascial pain).

The questions concerning the history and development of the headache problem may be useful in suggesting possible causes. For example, if a particular set of circumstances such as a holiday, or moving to a new job are associated with headache-free periods, and the presence of other events are associated with an increased frequency of headache attacks, the therapist may be able to develop some working hypotheses about the causes of the headaches. Close questioning is particularly helpful in cases where there has been quite a deal of fluctuation in the severity of the problem. It is especially useful to draw up a chronological table for such clients in order to identify more closely possible links between environmental events and headaches.

Questions concerning the frequency, duration and intensity of headaches will be useful in estimating the severity of the disorder. Of course, such estimation may be rather imprecise, and headache severity will ultimately be best assessed by the use of structured headache-recording assignments. The questions on headache features may require more explanation. The reader may well ask: what use does this detailed information have for the understanding and treatment of headache, especially if the distinctions between migraine and tension headache can be questioned? There are several reasons why detailed information should be gathered. First, the interviewer needs to be alert to gross deviations from the normal range of headache experiences. Such departures from a typical picture may suggest the need for further neurological, opthalmic or dental investigations. Second, a thorough assessment of the qualitative features of the headaches may lead to the use of more individually tailored self-monitoring devices. For instance, a patient who frequently experiences prodromal signs may be asked to monitor such occurrences in addition to the monitoring of headaches. Finally, there is some evidence that headache classification (based primarily on headache features) may be useful in predicting response to different types of interventions. For example, Blanchard *et al.* (1982) found that 52 per cent of tension-headache sufferers and 30 per cent of migraine-headache sufferers responded significantly to relaxation training. Admittedly, these findings are somewhat tentative, but it appears to be unwise at this stage to totally abandon the diagnostic distinction between migraine- and tension-headache patients.

Questions that revolve around the search for headache factors are the most problematic in an initial interview. Many patients have not closely examined their headache patterns, or may not be sufficiently aware of potential triggers to provide valid and reliable answers to such questions. It is often quite useful to discuss the concept of stress with the patient, pointing out that stressors may not necessarily be dramatic large-scale catastrophes, but are often relatively minor hassles and regularly occurring events. Some examples could be provided to illustrate the point, such as: being interrupted when trying to get some important work done, or having to deal with difficult people, or rushing to the supermarket at the last moment to buy ingredients for a dinner party, etc. Of course, some incidents from the person's accounts of his own headache attacks could be examined more closely. One could ask the client to provide details about the most recent headache attacks, although this kind of detailed analysis is best reserved until the second session, following an assignment to monitor the occurrence of any headaches. It may also be useful to administer a questionnaire designed to assess the occurrence of stressful life events such as the 'hassles scale' (Kanner *et al.*, 1981). This 117-item scale is designed to measure the occurrence of day-to-day hassles and frustrations. The hassles scale may be useful in the identification of idiosyncratic aversive or stressful events that may precede the onset of headaches. As previously noted, Bakal (1982) suggests that the headaches themselves may become a source of stress. Questions concerning this issue could be raised under the heading 'consequences' in the area under investigation listed later.

As discussed in Chapter 1, it is recommended that the therapist always obtains details of previous treatments and investigations. In particular, it may be worthwhile to explore the person's commitment to these treatments and the reasons for their failure, especially if such previous treatment involved some form of psychological therapy. From this information, the therapist may be alerted to likely problems in implementing the proposed intervention. It may also be useful to contact previous medical or psychological consultants if the client provides consent.

The interview

The following questions provide a guide to the areas of inquiry that may be useful in assessing clients who suffer from headaches.

General history

For how long have you been suffering from headaches?
Can you recall having headaches as a child?
What do you remember about them?
When did the headaches become a significant problem?
Have there been long periods without headaches? (*If so, obtain more details.*)
When? For how long? Under what circumstances?
Have headaches decreased when you have been on holiday, off work, etc.?
Do other family members suffer from headaches? (*You may need to specify various relations, e.g. mother, father, sister, children.*)

Frequency, duration, intensity

How often do headaches currently occur?
How many have there been in the last month?
What about during the last week — how many headaches have you had?
Is that the typical pattern at present? How long has that been the case?
Has there been a noticeable change in the frequency of headaches, e.g. are they increasing, decreasing or just remaining the same?
How long do your headaches typically last?
What is the longest one you can remember?
What is the shortest?
Has the duration of your headaches altered over time?
How severe is the pain? Do your headaches vary in severity?
Can you describe it for me?
Can you remember the worst headache that you have ever had?
What was that like?

Onset factors

What time of day do headaches typically start? (*Inquire into the range of the variation.*)
Do you ever wake with a headache at your normal waking time?
What time do you generally wake with a headache?
How often does this happen?
How do you feel when you wake with a headache?

Is your sleep interrupted by a headache in the middle of the night? How often?

Do you notice that your headaches occur on any particular days?

Do your headaches occur prior to particular activities or events? In particular, one should check out a number of common pre-headache stressors, e.g. interpersonal conflicts, non-assertion, dealing with difficult people, interactions with superiors at work, making decisions, giving directions to others, meeting deadlines, rushing, working long hours, working late, doing work that the person dislikes, etc.

Do they ever occur after particular activities have finished?

Do they ever occur while you are doing certain things?

Are there any foods or drinks that are often followed by a headache? (*Check specifically for chocolates, oranges, and alcohol.*)

Are there any other headache triggers? (*Check factors such as glare, reading, close-work, poor illumination.*)

Do you wear glasses? How long is it since these were changed?

How long is it since your last eye test? (*If the person reports visual difficulties and/or if there has been no recent opthalmological examination, such consultation should be recommended strongly.*)

Do you know if you have any dental problems?

Have you had any accidents or injuries that may be relevant to the headaches?

What do you think may be the cause of your headaches?

Are there any times when you notice that you don't get headaches? (*Check specifically about weekends, holidays and certain times of the day or year.*)

Headache features

Where do most headaches occur when the headache starts, e.g. the right forehead, behind the eye, in the neck, etc?

Does the pain move during headache attack? (*If so, obtain more details.*)

Is there a band or hat-like pressure?

How would you describe the headache?

Do you ever have any warning signs of a headache coming on?

What sort of signs do you get?

How long prior to the headache do these signs appear?

How long do they last?

Are your headaches ever accompanied by nausea or vomiting? It is also worthwhile checking what proportion of headaches are accompanied or preceded by various prodromal signs, nausea and vomiting, or other features.

Do you ever have these 'signs' without actually getting a headache?

Have you ever received a diagnosis of a specific headache type? What was the diagnosis, who made it and when?

Have the features of your headaches remained stable over time, or have there been variations? (*More details.*)

Do you think that you get more than one type of headache? (*If so, obtain more details of the distinctions that the person makes.*)

Check whether the headaches are ever accompanied by other features such as numbness, tears, running nose, deafness or other sensory disturbances, photophobia, sonophobia, constipation or diarrhoea.

Do you ever get that feeling of tenderness or soreness without an actual headache?

Consequences

What do you do when you have a headache attack? (*Have the person describe what typically happens from the time a headache is thought to be coming on, during the headache itself, and following the headache.*)

What do you think to yourself when you first notice the signs of a headache coming on?

Do you ever lie down when you're getting a headache? (*If so, obtain more details*).

Do you stop what you're doing and cancel plans? (*If so, obtain more details*).

How do other people react to you when you have a headache? (*Check reaction of spouse, close friends, children, etc.*)

Do you think you complain about your headaches much? (*If 'yes', obtain more details*).

To what extent are your leisure or work activities interfered with because of your headaches?

A recent or severe headache

It is often worthwhile to carefully investigate the details and circumstances of a recent or particularly severe headache. Such information often provides a richer source of information because of the recency of the occasion or because of the particularly strong memories of an especially bad headache. You could proceed as follows:

When was the last headache that you had?

Let's go over this headache in a bit more detail. What time did it start? How long did it last?
How bad was it, compared with your other headaches?
Can you describe how it felt?
Where was the pain located?
Can you remember how it came on and what you were doing at the time?
What had you been doing prior to that in the day?
What were your plans for the rest of the day?
What did you do when you had the headache?
Did you lie down?
Did you go home from work or stop doing what you were doing?
Did you take any medication? What sort? How much?
Did you tell anyone that you had a headache? Who? What did they say?
How did the headache go away?
What do you think might have caused that particular headache?

One might repeat this set of questions with respect to a number of headaches that have been experienced recently.

Prior treatment/investigations

What treatments are you currently using to help with the headaches? (*Check the names of specific drugs, the number/amount taken, the time at which it was taken in relation to headache or prodromal phase, the effects, how long has the person been taking the various medications, etc.*)
Are you taking any tablets for any other reason? (*If so, obtain more details.*)
Which treatments have you tried previously? When? For how long? What effects did they have?
Have you had any experience with relaxation training or similar procedures? When? For how long? What were the effects? What did the relaxation actually consist of?
What medical checks, surgery, etc. have you had? When? What were the results? (*Check especially for detailed neurological examination. Dental and opthalmological investigations may also provide useful information.*)

Other aspects

The questions outlined in the preceding section deal specifically with the headache problem. Of course, the interviewer should be alert to the presence of other problems. The assessment of any experiences of anxiety and tension would be the most relevant area of inquiry (also see Chapter 2). Apart from a general assessment of tension/anxiety problems, it may be useful to assess the extent to which the person is troubled by feelings of depression. Several researchers have noted the relationship between depression and headache, although the direction of causality, if indeed there is one, is not clear. Diamond (1983) argues that it is characteristic of these depression-related headaches that the person wakes with a headache or develops a headache very early in the day, and that the headaches often appear during periods of rest such as weekends or holidays. It should also be noted here that Moss, McClure, Jackson & Lombardo (1987) have shown that some individuals are prone to early-morning headache after sleeping for an additional two hours beyond their normal sleep time. For those cases in which depression is suspected to be involved, it may be possible to derive specific hypotheses about such depression – headache relationships and to develop appropriate individual treatment programmes. The reader is referred to Chapter 3 for a discussion of the assessment of depression.

Predictors of response

There has been very little study of the predictors of response to behavioural treatments for headache. However, a few indications have emerged from the literature to date. Patients with relatively continuous headache have poorer outcomes compared with patients with discrete headache attacks. It has also been found that depressed patients have a poorer prognosis than non-depressed headache sufferers (Jacob, Turner, Szekely & Eidelman, 1983). Finally, Blanchard and his colleagues have provided predictor equations to indicate the likely response to treatment based on psychological (Blanchard *et al.*, 1982) and physiological factors (Blanchard *et al.*, 1983). Consideration of the above prognostic factors may alert the therapist to potentially difficult clients. Such information may be useful in suggesting alterations that may need to be made to a treatment programme. For example, it may be useful to intervene more specifically on mood problems with a depressive headache client.

Behavioural assessment of headache

The most commonly employed headache-assessment device

Table 8.1: *Headache-recording form*

Please indicate the time when the headache started and finished on the form, and rate the severity of the pain on the scale from 0 to 5.

0 = no pain, 1 = a little pain, barely noticeable, 2 = mild pain, 3 = moderate pain, 4 = very bad pain, 5 = severe pain

Time headache commenced ....

Time headache finished ....

Severity of headache (at worst)...

Were there any other sensations other than the pain (e.g. nausea, vomiting, visual disturbance, etc)?

If so, give details ....

....

....

....

Did you take any medication? Type .... Dosage ....

What were you doing at the time the headache started?.................................

....

....

....

consists of a headache-monitoring form such as the one contained in Table 8.1. This kind of procedure can be employed to produce a number of different headache measures:

1. Number of headaches in a specified period.
2. Average (and peak) of intensity.
3. Average duration.
4. Number of headache-free days.

A headache index, combining frequency, intensity and duration can also be calculated using a method originally described by Budzynski, Stoyva, Adler & Mullaney (1973).

A headache-monitoring form can be employed as a measure of treatment outcome, and as a means for identifying temporal or other patterns of headache occurrence. Patients can be asked to record any possible antecedent or consequent events on the headache-monitoring form once they have been trained to identify such events in the therapy sessions. Consumption of medication can also be recorded as an additional index of changes during treatment. Of course, such self-report devices are open to problems such as faking, response bias and so forth. The psychometric properties of headache-monitoring devices have not been examined extensively, although the data available suggests adequate validity (Blanchard, Andrasik, Neff, Jurish & O'Keefe, 1981).

Several issues may arise in the use of headache-monitoring forms. Occasionally, clients will return to sessions complaining that the monitoring is making them worse. It is important to examine whether there is validity to this claim, to check whether the person has an accurate perception of the monitoring task itself and to stress the importance of the self-monitoring as a collaborative effort to obtain details of the headache attacks that may be useful in therapy. Sometimes, it appears that clients misconstrue the nature of the task, and become rather obsessive about the regularity of checking for head pain throughout the day. It may be best to preselect certain recording times, such as 8.00 a.m., midday, 4.00 p.m., 8.00 p.m. and bedtime for such individuals (even less regularly if necessary). Some redesign of the task or the actual monitoring form may be helpful for particular clients.

Apart from the assessment of headache frequency, intensity and duration, the therapist may find it useful to assess the occurrence of headache-related cognitions. Bakal (1982) has produced the 'headache assessment questionnaire', which consists of 48 statements reflective of the thoughts and feelings that are frequently experienced during a headache attack, such as 'I wonder if I'll have to cancel any plans', 'I feel guilty about having another headache', and 'This headache is driving me crazy'. Administration of this questionnaire may be helpful in the identification of specific headache-related cognitions that would become targets of intervention in cognitive theory.

The therapist may find it useful to conduct physiological assessment of headache patients. EMG recordings from a number of sites in the head and neck region, measures of vascular activity or digital skin-temperature recordings would represent the most useful assessment in the physiological mode. A complete discussion of physiological recording is beyond the scope of the present text, but the interested reader could consult Gaardner and Montgomery (1977) for further information.

Thompson and Figueroa (1983) have proposed a very interesting method for combining the information from the various modes of headache assessment in a type of profile analysis. They recommend the routine collection of data from five sources: questionnaire, self-monitoring, musculo-skeletal, vascular and autonomic. The questionnaire and self-monitoring sources could be constructed to provide information on the importance of perceived physiological aspects, cognitive components and environmental stressors. The musculo-skeletal, vascular and autonomic recordings could be obtained during (1) a non-headache period; (2) the development of a headache; (3) the occurrence of a headache; and (4) the presentation of a series of laboratory stress situations, preferably designed to simulate real-life stressors. This kind of multimodal assessment requires access to sophisticated laboratory equipment, although less ambitious variants may be devised. The general principle that underlies this thorough assessment seems to be particularly worthy of further investigation, as the resulting profiles may prove to be useful in the selection of treatment procedures that are tailored more to the needs of individual clients.

Treatment

There are numerous medical and psychological treatments for headache. Medical treatments include such medications as aspirin, methysergide, ergotamine, anxiolytics and antidepressants. Much medical treatment of headache is palliative (i.e. designed to abort the headache once it has started, or once the prodromal signs have appeared.) Some medications, such as antidepressant drugs and methysergide substances, may be also prescribed to be taken on a regular basis as a prophylactic procedure. In either case, patients with chronic headache are often prescribed large amounts of medication in the hope of providing some relief. The disadvantages of such treatments are fairly obvious. Headaches may still occur with such frequency that the individual continues to suffer considerable pain and interference with leisure and work activities. In addition, serious medical consequences, such as liver and kidney disease, may be incurred as a result of long periods of intensive medication. The aim of most psychological treatments is to prevent the occurrence of the headache through the use of various stress-management procedures such as relaxation (Bernstein & Borkovec, 1973), biofeedback (Budzynski *et al.*, 1973) or cognitive therapy (Holroyd & Andrasik, 1978; Holroyd, Andrasik & Westbrook, 1977).

For a discussion of medical and psychological treatments, the reader is referred to Bakal (1982), which includes a manual for conducting cognitive-behaviour therapy with headache sufferers. Blanchard and Andrasik (1985) have also produced a very comprehensive manual for the management of headaches. The relaxation-training manual of Bernstein and Borkovec (1973) is also very useful as a general guide to the use of relaxation procedures. For discussion of the treatment of sleep-related and TMJ induced headaches, the reader is advised to consult Moss (in press). Reviews of the headache-treatment literature are presented by Blanchard, Ahles & Shaw (1979), Blanchard & Andrasik (1982), Blanchard, Andrasik, Ahles, Teders & O'Keefe (1980) and Bakal (1982).

9
Substance Abuse

Introduction

There are two main types of substance use problems that practitioners will encounter. The first set are the acute problems that occur during intoxication or withdrawal, including psychoses that may be triggered by the use of the substance. These are detailed within the DSM-III-R (American Psychiatric Association, 1987) section on organic mental disorders and do not form the primary focus of this chapter. The second set refer to long-term problems and are classified by DSM-III-R in the section on psychoactive substance use disorders. The classification distinguishes two types of disorder: (1) psychoactive substance dependence; and (2) psychoactive substance abuse. Substance dependence is seen as a more serious form of disorder, and is characterised by at least three out of nine features: (1) a person often takes the drug in larger amounts or over a longer period than was intended; (2) he or she has a persistent desire or has had one or more attempts to cut down or control substance use; (3) he or she spends a great deal of time in activities to obtain the substance, to use it or to recover from its effects; (4) he or she shows frequent intoxication or withdrawal symptoms when expected to fulfil social or occupational obligations, or when substance use is physically hazardous; (5) important social, occupational, or recreational activity is given up or reduced because it was incompatible with the use of the drug; (6) there is continued use despite a persistent social, occupational or physical problem that is caused by, or exacerbated by use of the substance; (7) there is a marked tolerance, where a markedly increased amount (at least 50 per cent more) is required to achieve intoxication or the desired effect, or there is markedly diminished effect from the continued use of the same amount; and *except for cannabis, hallucinogens and phencyclidine (PCP)*: (8) withdrawal symptoms occur; and (9) the person often takes the drug to relieve or avoid withdrawal symptoms. Substance abuse is coded when the person does not show sufficient features for dependence, but does not exhibit either feature (6) above (continued use despite a persistent substance-related problem), or recurrent use in situations when use is hazardous (after feature 4 above). In both cases, some of these features must have persisted over a month, or occurred repeatedly over some longer period.

The revision represents a substantial improvement over DSM-III, in that it now includes a wider range of features characterising dependence, and also allows a simple rating of severity based on the number of observed features and the degree of impairment in social or occupational functioning. However, the categorisation still suffers from imprecision in terms such as 'recurrent', 'persistent', 'frequent' and 'a great deal of time'. Further difficulties are created by the assessment of social or occupational problems, since these are partially dependent on the subjective reactions of others in the person's social network — reactions that may vary across observers and over time. Consistent additional criteria will be required to ensure a reliable judgment by interviewers. More importantly, criteria for dependence combine physiological and psychosocial problems that may be better kept separate. The interview in this chapter may be used to decide whether a person fulfils the criteria for DSM-III-R, but this is not its primary focus. Rather, the emphasis is placed on a functional assessment that may be applied to designing interventions.

Commonly abused substances are usually classed into depressants, stimulants and hallucinogens. Depressants are substances that reduce central nervous system activity, such as alcohol, barbiturates, benzodiazepines, narcotic analgesics and many inhalants. Stimulants produce signs of increased arousal and include caffeine, nicotine, amphetamines and cocaine. As the name suggests, hallucinogens provoke perceptual distortions. Some examples are LSD, mescaline, PCP ('angel dust') and psilocybin ('magic mushrooms'). Cannabis shows properties of a depressant and at larger doses, it is also hallucinogenic. Many other substances have biphasic effects: alcohol, for example, induces an initial increase in heart rate and blood pressure before producing sedation. These transient effects may be important sources of immediate reinforcement for substance use. Consumption of multiple drugs can also produce interactional effects. For example, cocaine is often taken to modify the sedative effects of heroin, but, in fact, both substances depress the respiratory centre. A user may inadvertently precipitate respiratory failure through using the substances in combination.

A detailed description of substance effects and risks lies outside the scope of this chapter. Readers are referred to a general view such as Madden (1979) and to publications on individual substances such as Eastman (1984) on alcohol, Hughes & Hatsukami (1986) and Krasnegor (1979) on tobacco, James & Crosbie (1987) on caffeine, Institute of Medicine (1982) on cannabis, Grabowski (1984) and Gawin and Kleber (1986) on cocaine, Allison & Jerrom (1984) and Watson (1980) on solvents and Kornblith (1981) on other substances.

On the surface, it may seem odd to combine the assessment of such a diverse set of substance-abuse problems into a single chapter. However, in recent years, there has been a growing awareness of the psychological similarities between the processes involved in the abuse of different substances (e.g. Miller, 1980; Solomon, 1980), and a number of psychological models have been advanced that relate to substance abuse in general (Blane & Leonard, 1987; Brownell, Marlatt, Lichtenstein & Wilson, 1986; Hull, 1981; Ludwig & Wikler, 1984; MacRae, Scoles & Siegel, 1987; Orford, 1985; Prochaska & Di Climente, 1983; Solomon, 1980; Steele, Southwick & Pagano, 1986). Reviews are presented by Wilson (1987) and Saunders and Allsop (1987).

A model presented by Marlatt and Gordon (1985) has provoked considerable interest among practitioners. This model focuses on the processes involved in relapse. Former users often place themselves in situations where they are at high risk of relapse (Marlatt & Gordon, 1985). Once in the situation, they are especially likely to use the substance if they have poor skills in dealing with the situation, have low self-efficacy about resisting substance use (Bandura, 1977b, 1982), and have positive expectancies about the effects of the substance. If they do succumb to temptation, people who are committed to an abstinence goal experience an 'abstinence violation effect' that consists of cognitive dissonance, associated negative emotion and a reduction in self-efficacy about their future control of substance use. This effect predisposes to a full relapse. Initial research supports the model (Curry, Marlatt & Gordon, 1987) and suggests that application of the model to problem solving and skills training may be very productive (Chaney, O'Leary & Marlatt, 1978; cf. Supnick & Coletti, 1984). The interview described below encourages an assessment of features from Marlatt and Gordon's model that appear to be especially important.

Although a number of psychological theories of substance abuse are now available, twentieth-century conceptions of substance abuse have been dominated by a disease model, particularly in the area of alcoholism (e.g. Jellinek, 1960). Some support for somatic factors is provided by a growing literature that attests the role of genetic factors in the causation of alcoholism and other substance abuse (Braude & Chao, 1986; Schuckitt, 1987). However, the disease model is often pushed much further. In its pure form, such a model is clearly antithetical to a cognitive-behavioural explanation of substance abuse, since it discounts the role of environmental or skill factors in its maintenance (cf. Heather & Robertson, 1983). The disease model has also been associated with the view that total and permanent abstinence is the only appropriate treatment goal for alcoholics, because of the severe craving and loss of control that they show. While the insistence on abstinence has attracted trenchant criticism over recent years (e.g. Chase, Salzberg & Palotai, 1984; Heather & Robertson, 1983), the evidence suggests that an abstinence goal may be preferable for clients with severe dependence (Chase *et al.*, 1984; Heather & Robertson, 1983). Whichever view is taken about the treatment goal that should be adopted or the extent that predispositional factors enter into the development of substance abuse, a functional analysis is required to ascertain the current maintaining conditions and the strategies that should be adopted to deal with the problem. The interview below is intended to meet this need.

The interview

Because of the sensitive nature of the information being obtained in this interview, it is particularly important to obtain the person's trust and to clarify rules of confidentiality before beginning. Special difficulties may be posed by disclosure of criminal offences by the client, or by situations where a report to a court may be requested. Note also that the recent memory of alcoholics may have been affected by their substance use, and recollections may need to be confirmed from other sources.

Throughout the interview, the questions refer to 'use of the substance'. Substitute a phrase that is appropriate to the particular substance, e.g. 'drinking', 'shooting up smack/heroin', 'taking speed', etc. The questions assume that the interviewer already knows the person's age, marital status and employment history (see Chapter 1).

Identification of target substances

If the person has been referred for assessment regarding a specific substance:

In this interview, I want to talk to you about your use of substance X. What can you tell me about it? Why do you think you have been referred?

If the referral is less specific:

In this interview, I want to talk to you about alcohol and other drugs. First of all, I want you to tell me which ones you have ever used in the past — coffee or tea, alcohol, sleeping tablets or tranquillizers, amphetamines ('*uppers*') or 'poppers' (*volatile nitrites*), or any other tablets or cigarettes, cigars or snuff? Have you ever used marihuana ('*grass*'/'*pot*') or hashish ('*hash*') or cocaine ('*coke*', '*crack*') or anything like LSD or 'magic mushrooms' (*psilocybin*)? Have you sniffed anything, like glue or gas/petrol or used heroin ('*smack*', '*horse*'), morphine, methadone or cough syrups or anything else?

For each substance that the person has used in the past, ask:

Have you used the substance in the past three months? How often?

Initially, focus on the substance that seems to represent the most serious potential problem.

Consumption

Questions about consumption often ask about typical usage levels. This type of data is prone to error because it relies not only on clients being able to recall a representative selection of consumption occasions, but also asks them to estimate an average (cf. Gregson & Stacey, 1982). The approach taken here is to examine the most recent occasions and obtain an estimate of their typicality.

When was the last day you used it?

If there are different types of the substance:

What exactly did you have?

The person's replies can be used to assess the dosage used. In the case of alcohol, refer to Table 9.1 for the amount of ethanol in

Table 9.1: *Alcohol content of alcoholic beverages*

Drink (% alcohol by vol.)	Quantity	Alcohol content[1]
Regular beer (4–5% alcohol)[2]	285 ml (10 oz glass)*	11.3 gms
	340 ml (12 oz bottle)	13.4 gms
	375 ml (13 oz can)	14.8 gms
	425 ml (15 oz glass)	16.8 gms
Wine (10–12% alcohol)	114 ml (4 oz glass)*	10.8 gms
	750 ml (26.4 oz bottle)	71.1 gms
	1000 ml (35.2 oz bottle)	94.8 gms
Sherry, port, vermouth (18–20% alcohol)	60 ml (2 oz)*	9.5 gms
	750 ml (26.4 oz bottle)	118.5 gms
Spirits (40% alcohol)[3]	30 ml (1 oz)*	9.5 gms
	375 ml (13.2 oz bottle)	118.5 gms
	750 ml (26.4 oz bottle)	237.0 gms
	1135 ml (40 oz bottle)	358.7 gms

Notes: *Closest quantity to a standard drink (10 gms alcohol). Note that glasses may differ in size: for example many wine glasses hold 5 oz or more.

1. The volume of absolute alcohol in mls is calculated by multiplying the volume of the drink by the upper estimate of % alcohol in the table. To derive the mass in gms, this figure is multiplied by the specific gravity of ethanol (0.79). This calculation method may lead to an overestimation of intake where the alcohol content is less than the upper limit in the table.

2. The alcohol content of beers and ales varies across breweries and over time. This is the approximate content of regular beer in Australia or the United States, and of light ale in Britain (Mellor, 1970). In Britain, bitter beer is about 3.5%, stout is about 5.5% and strong ale can be as high as 8% (Mellor, 1970). Calculate the amount of ethanol in low-alcohol beers by relating their percentage alcohol to regular beer: e.g. a 10 oz glass of 2.2% beer has $(2.2/5) \times 11.3 = 5$ gms alcohol.

3. This is equivalent to 70° proof in the UK, 80° proof in the US.

common drinks. For street drugs, it may be difficult to estimate the amount consumed because of variation in the extent they are diluted. For example, heroin is commonly diluted to 15–20%, but a purity as high as 90% may sometimes be obtained. If there are different routes of administration for the substance (e.g. sniffing, shooting up, taking tablets):

How did you take it?

If it was taken intravenously:

Did you sterilise the needle? Did any other people share the needle?

People who intend to continue using the substance may respond to information and skills training to reduce their risk of infection.

How much did you have? Over what period?

Since heavy consumption is generally seen as undesirable, clients may often understate their intake (Midanik, 1982). Conversely, narcotic-dependent clients may sometimes overstate their usage in order to maximise the dosage of methadone. A partial solution to this problem is to look at other indicators of dosage, such as cost per week and withdrawal signs. As a guide, the average daily amount of heroin for a street user is about 30–60 mg (Senay, 1983).

Even when these influences are not operating, consumption is often difficult to estimate. Not only may the intoxication interfere with accurate monitoring, but attention will often be focused on conversations or other events. Situational features such as a waiter continually replenishing a glass or a group sharing a joint of marihuana may further complicate the task. Sometimes there are social cues that will help: for example, when each member of the group takes turns in buying drinks, the number of people by the number of turns provides the amount. Sometimes the total number of bottles or packets or the amount of money used to buy the substance can be estimated. If possible, cross-verify using different estimation methods.

Details about consumption can be used to determine maximum levels of the substance in the body. For example, alcohol is metabolised at a rate of about 1.5 standard drinks per hour in a healthy person. Given the person's weight and gender, data about the amount of alcohol and the consumption period can be used to estimate blood-alcohol levels, provided we assume an average rate of absorption and metabolism and a stable rate of consumption. Tables in Miller & Munoz (1982, pp. 8–11) give approximate values.

> When was the previous day you used the substance? How much did you have then?
>
> So the last two times you used the substance were . . . days apart — was that fairly typical? (In what way did it differ?)
>
> What about the amounts? You had . . . on these occasions over about . . . hours/day — was that the same as usual?

Derive a quantity/frequency estimate using the most recent amount divided by the last recalled interval between occasions (Gregson & Stacey, 1982), modifying this estimate only if there is good reason to view it as atypical.

Loss of control and binges

> Do you sometimes find that you are having more of the

substance than you meant to, or use it for a longer time than you intended?
(*If yes*:) How often does that happen?
Have you ever gone on a binge, i.e. used the substance almost continuously for more than a day, or until it ran out?
(*If yes*:) When was the last one? How did it start? How long did it last? How did it finish? When was the previous time? Does it typically occur every _____ (*interval*)?

Changes in consumption and development of tolerance

Has the amount you use changed over the past year?
(*If no*:) How long have you been using that amount?
(*If it has increased*:) Do you need to use more of the substance to get the same effects as you used to, say, a year ago? How much more do you have to use?
(*If it is the same*:) Does that amount give the same effects as it did a year ago?
(*If no*:) In what way has the effect changed?

Stimuli

I'd like to have some more information about the situations where you use the substance. (*If the person is using an illegal drug you may need to clarify confidentiality.*)
Going back to the last time you used the substance. Where were you? What was happening? Was anyone else there?
(*If yes*:) Were they using the substance? What were you doing before that?
How about the previous time you used the substance — where were you, etc?
Are those the kinds of situation where you usually use the substance? Do you use it at other times or places or with other people?

Immediate consequences

The last time you used the substance, how did it make you feel?
Have you ever had unpleasant effects from the substance? (*Look for unwanted physical symptoms, cognitive/perceptual effects (e.g. loss of concentration, memory problems, hallucinations, delusions), affect changes (e.g. anger, fear, depression).*)

Withdrawal

The last time you used the substance, how did you feel after-

wards/the next morning? (*Look for withdrawal signs of the particular substance* (DSM-III-R, 1987).)
Have you ever had withdrawal effects from the substance? Have you ever used the substance to get rid of these effects, or used it first thing in the morning?
(*If yes*:) When was the last time and the time before that? Is that about how frequently you usually do that?
Have you ever used any other drug to cope with the effects when you stop using? (*If yes, ascertain how often the person does this, and whether they use the substance at other times.*)

Medical consequences

Have you had any accidents or injuries in the past year?
(*If yes:*) Have any of these occurred after you used the substance? (*Physical injury is a common outcome of substance abuse (Skinner, Holt, Schuller, Roy & Israel, 1984; Tinklenberg, 1973).*)
Have you had any illnesses over the past year?
Do you have any current health problems? (*Note any problems that may be related to the substance use or to the person's lifestyle.*)
How is your appetite at the moment? Have you gained or lost any weight recently? What have you eaten today? Yesterday? Is that the usual amount you would eat? Have you ever missed meals when you are using the substance?
Have you ever received medical treatment because of your substance use? Have you ever overdosed on the substance so that it made you ill? Has a doctor ever advised you to stop using the substance or to reduce the amount you use? Why?

Social consequences

Has anyone been criticising your use of the substance? Has this caused any arguments?
Have you ever used the substance secretly? Has that happened recently?
Has your social or family life been affected by your use of the substance in any other way?
Have you ever lost friends or had a relationship break up over it? Have you gained friends through your substance use? Are they users too?
(*If the person is currently employed*:) Have you noticed any effects on your work? Have you gone to work when you have been feeling the effects of the substance? Have you been late or had any time off work because of your substance use?

(*If yes*:) How often do these things happen? Have you ever lost a job because of them?

Changes in activities

Are there any interests or activities that you are less involved in now than in the past?
(*If yes*:) Are there times when you don't do these things because of your substance use?
Are there any activities or interest that you have become involved in?
(*If yes*:) Do any of those involve using the substance?

These questions may be supplemented by analysing responses to a 'pleasant events schedule' (MacPhillamy & Lewinsohn, 1982).

How much time did you spend thinking about the substance yesterday?
Did you spend any time arranging to get the substance?
Was that a typical amount of time?

Financial consequences

Can you estimate how much you spent on your habit last week?
Is that a typical amount?

Users will often find this hard to estimate, and answers will often be grossly inaccurate. When a figure can be derived, it gives a further indication of the amount being consumed.

How do you support your habit? Does finding that money produce problems?

Legal consequences

Have you ever had any legal problems or fights when you have been using the substance? (*If yes*:) Tell me about that.
Have you ever been arrested for driving under the influence? (*If yes*:) How many times has that happened?
(*In the case of alcohol*:) Do you know what your blood-alcohol level was? (*Blood-alcohol levels provide convergent data on past consumption.*)
Have you ever had any other legal problems, e.g. any arrests for dealing, or stealing to support your habit?

Others with problems

Has anyone you know had a problem with alcohol or other drugs, e.g. any of your relatives?
(*If the answer is yes in either case*:) What sort of problem was that? Did they try to do something about it? What happened?

Answers will provide information about possible environmental or genetic influences as well as revealing the person's views about drug problems and their solutions.

Perceived dissatisfaction, previous attempts

Do you think you have a problem with your use of the substance? (*If yes*:) In what way? How long have you felt it was a problem? (*If no*:) Have you ever thought you would prefer to use the substance less, or even stop altogether? How often do you think that? Does anyone else think you have a problem with the substance? Why is that?

Have you tried to stop or cut down in the past?

(*If yes*:) How often have you tried? When was the last time? What prompted you to try? What methods did you use? How long did it last? What situation were you in when you started using it again?

What is the longest time you have tried to stay off (the substance)? (*If the longest was not the last attempt, obtain further details.*)

The fact that a person has tried to restrict his consumption implies a past dissatisfaction with the substance use. Information about past attempts also helps to clarify present motivation and confidence about being able to control substance use, alerting the interviewer to situations that may predispose relapse in the future. Negative emotional states, interpersonal conflict and social pressure commonly pose a high risk for relapse (Chaney *et al.*, 1978; Shiffman, 1982).

Have you ever tried to get help for your substance use?

(*If yes*:) When was that? What was it? What happened?

Present intentions

If the person expresses current discontent about his substance use:

You said that you are unhappy about your use of the substance at the moment. What do you want to do about it? (*Clarify the person's preferred goal, and whether he is seeking assistance.*)

(*If the person requires treatment*:) What sort of treatment do you think would help you?

Perceived effects of stopping or cutting down

Are you worried about any effects you would experience if you stopped using the substance altogether?

Fears of withdrawal may require treatment before the person is willing to stop or cut down. Fear of withdrawal from narcotics is particularly common (Hall, 1984). People who contemplate stopping smoking may be concerned about weight gain (Hall, Ginsberg & Jones, 1986).

What would you miss most about using the substance? (*Look for perceived cognitive, affective and social benefits from using the drug.*)

What do you think would be the best thing about stopping/cutting down?

As well as assessing the problem, this interview should foster the person's motivation for reduction where appropriate. Answers to the question will also provide ideas for reinforcers of behaviour change.

Social support for change

(*If the person is living with others*:) Do the people you live with use the substance? If you tried to stop/cut down, how would your family and friends react? Is there anyone who would give you support? What would they do? Is there anyone who would be pressuring you to use the substance again? What would they do?

Are there any situations where you never use the substance?

Are there any other situations in which it would be relatively easy to stop or cut down? What situations would be hardest?

Answers are likely to uncover subjective loss of control, and situations where craving or ruminations about the substance are most severe. If self-control training is planned, a more detailed assessment of potential inconsistent activities and a hierarchy of situations may be required. The 'cues for drinking questionnaire' (Rankin, Stockwell & Hodgson, 1982) may assist in ranking problem situations for alcohol use, and adaptions may be attempted for other drugs.

Other substance use

If the substance is not available, do you use something else?

Check particularly for the use of more risky alternatives to the substance, such as nonbeverage alcohol.

Have you ever used more than one drug at once?

Many people asking for substance-abuse treatment are multiple drug users (e.g. Istvan & Matarazzo, 1984; Perera, Tulley & Jenner, 1987). A further interview will be required to assess the use of other substances that constitute a significant problem.

Other problems

A large proportion of people seeking treatment for substance use also have a range of other problems such as depression and anxiety disorders (Hesselbrock, Meyer & Keener, 1985). A separate assessment interview relating to these problems may be necessary to ascertain whether additional treatment is required.

Specific assessment instruments

Self-report screening measures

Screening instruments for alcohol and other drug problems may be applied before undertaking a detailed interview. Perhaps the best known of these is the 'Michigan alcoholism screening test' (MAST; Selzer, 1971; Selzer, Gomberg & Nordhoff, 1979). The MAST was originally a 25-item interview instrument. Modifications include shorter versions (e.g. BMAST; Pokorney, Miller & Kaplan, 1972; cf. Kaplan, Pokorney, Kanes & Lively, 1974; Mm-MAST; Kristenson & Trell, 1982) and self-administration (SAAST; Morse & Hurt, 1979; Hurt, Morse & Swenson, 1980; Swenson & Morse, 1975). Reliability data on the MAST is reported by Skinner & Sheu (1982) and Jacobson (1984) provides a review. The 'drug abuse screening test' (DAST; Skinner, 1982) represents an adaptation of the MAST to detect abuse of a wide range of drugs.

The CAGE (Mayfield, McLeod & Hall, 1974; cf. Ewing, 1984) consists of four questions: (1) Have you ever felt you should *cut down* your drinking? (2) Have people *annoyed* you by criticising your drinking? (3) Have you ever felt bad or *guilty* about your drinking? and (4) Have you ever had a drink first thing in the morning to steady your nerves, or to get rid of a hangover (*eye-opener*)? This test is highly sensitive to severe forms of alcohol abuse, but is less successful with milder problems. Another simple test is the 'trauma questionnaire' (Skinner *et al.*, 1984) which asks five questions about adult injuries and is especially successful in detecting alcohol problems when used in conjunction with biochemical markers. Other scales to screen for alcohol problems include the 'MacAndrew scale' (MacAndrew, 1965; cf. Preng & Clopton, 1986), the 'Alcadd test' (Ornstein, 1976), the 'adolescent alcohol involvement scale' (Mayer & Filstead, 1979; Moberg, 1983) and the 'spare time activities questionnaire' (Wilkins, 1974; see also the 'Clydebank questionnaire', Saunders & Kershaw, 1978, 1980).

Self-report measures of dependence

Screening measures are primarily concerned with identifying people who have problems with substance use. In the present section, we examine scales that are designed to assess the degree of problem. Tests of alcohol dependence achieve special importance because highly dependent people are less likely to have a controlled drinking outcome (Hodgson, Stockwell, Rankin & Edwards, 1978; Polich, Armour & Braiker, 1980). The most commonly used tests of alcohol dependence are the 'severity of alcohol dependence questionnaire' (SADQ; Stockwell, Hodgson, Edwards, Taylor & Rankin, 1979; Stockwell, Murphy & Hodgson, 1983) and the 'alcohol dependence scale' (ADS; Skinner & Allen, 1982). Each of these has sound psychometric characteristics. The SADQ is now administered as a 20-item questionnaire and places heavy emphasis on withdrawal symptoms. Scores are significantly correlated with medication required during detoxification (Cooney, Meyer, Kaplan & Baker, 1986). The ADS is a 25-item questionnaire derived from the 'alcohol use inventory' (AUI; Horn, Wanberg & Foster, 1974; Wanberg, Horn & Foster, 1977).

Other scales include the 'short alcohol dependence data questionnaire' (SADD; Raistrick, Dunbar & Davidson, 1983), which aims to increase discriminative power in the mild to moderate range, the 'Rand dependence scale' (Polich *et al.*, 1980) and the 'Edinburgh alcohol dependence schedule' (EADS; Chick, 1980). The type or degree of alcohol problem is also assessed by the 'drinking behaviour interview' (Shelton, Hollister & Gocka, 1969; Schultz, Kelley, Overall & Hollister, 1985), the 'addiction severity index' (ASI; Erdlen, McLellan, La Porte *et al.*, 1978; McLellan, Luborsky, Woody & O'Brien, 1980; McLellan *et al.*, 1985), the 'last six months of drinking questionnaire' and the 'last 30 days of drinking questionnaire' (Hesselbrook, Babor, Hesselbrook, Meyer & Workman, 1983; cf. Cooney *et al.*, 1986) and the 'Missouri alcoholism severity scale' (Evenson, 1986; Evenson, Holland & Cho, 1979).

For narcotic dependence, the 'severity of opiate dependence questionnaire' (SODQ; Sutherland, Edwards, Taylor, Phillips, Gossop & Brady, 1986) has recently been adapted from the SADQ. Although initial data are encouraging, further evidence of its utility is required. Information based on other measures suggests that dependence on narcotics has less relationship with outcome than does alcohol dependence (Babor, Cooney & Laverman,

1987). Similarly, nicotine dependence is often measured by the 'nicotine tolerance questionnaire' of Fagerstrom (1982), but some recent evidence queries whether this questionnaire consistently predicts outcome (e.g. Hall, Tunstall, Rugg, Jones & Benowitz, 1985).

Self-efficacy measures

Applying a concept developed by Bandura (1977b, 1982), self-efficacy measures ask the person about his capability in abstaining or controlling substance use in specific situations, and can be used to predict relapse and develop targets for skill training. Measures have been developed for tobacco smoking (Best & Hakstian, 1978; Condiotte & Lichtenstein, 1981; Di Climente, 1981; Godding & Glasgow, 1985; Yates & Thain, 1985) and for alcohol (Rist & Watzl, 1983), and may be adapted for use with other substances. Consistent with self-efficacy theory, ratings are strongly correlated with outcome over three to six months, but the relationship decreases over longer follow-up periods (McIntyre, Lichtenstein & Mermelstein, 1983).

A measure that is probably related to self-efficacy is the 'cues for drinking questionnaire' (Rankin, Stockwell & Hodgson, 1982), which asks how frequently subjects would drink if faced with particular situations. Negative moods are more important than withdrawal for moderately dependent persons. This effect disappears in more severe dependence.

Substance expectancy measures

These scales provide information about the effects that the person expects the substance to have on him. 'Alcohol expectancy questionnaires' have been developed by Brown, Goldman, Inn & Anderson (1982), Christianson, Goldman & Inn (1982), Donovan & Marlatt (1980), Southwick, Steele, Marlatt & Lindell (1981) and Young & Knight (1986). Fears about methadone withdrawal can be assessed on the 'detoxification fear survey schedule' of Milby, Gurwitch, Wiebe, Ling, McLellan & Woody (1986).

Table 9.2: *Sample self-monitoring form for alcohol*

Drinking tally For week beginning..........................

Please fill out this form as soon as possible after a drinking occasion and at least once each day.

Complete a new section each time the situation changes, even if this occurs several times a day.

Day ....What drink ....Size............How many............

Began...........am/pm What drink.............Size............How many............

Ended...........am/pm What drink.............Size............How many............

Where were you?...........................Who were you with?...........................

What happened before? ....

What happened next?...

Day ....What drink ....Size............How many............

Began...........am/pm What drink.............Size............How many............

Ended...........am/pm What drink.............Size............How many............

Where were you?...........................Who were you with?...........................

What happened before? ....

What happened next?...

Day ....What drink ....Size............How many............

Began...........am/pm What drink.............Size............How many............

Ended...........am/pm What drink.............Size............How many............

Where were you?...........................Who were you with?...........................

What happened before? ....

What happened next?...

Self-monitoring

When abstinence is beginning immediately, it may not be possible to obtain any self-monitoring data. Other clients may be asked to self-monitor consumption over one to two weeks. Sample monitoring forms for alcohol and cigarette consumption are shown in Tables 9.2 and 9.3. These forms can be adapted for use with other substances. Self-monitoring provides data on consumption, stimuli and reinforcers that is less subject to recall than information derived from the interview as long as it is completed

Table 9.3: *Sample self-monitoring form for cigarettes*

Cigarette tally For week beginning ______________

For each hour of the day, place a cross on the page every time you have a cigarette.

Day ....

10																								
9																								
8																								
7																								
6																								
5																								
4																								
3																								
2																								
1																								
	1	2	3	4	5	6	7	8	9	10	11	12	1	2	3	4	5	6	7	8	9	10	11	12
						am						noon						pm						

At the end of the day, notice the period when you had the most cigarettes.

Where were you? ....

Who were you with? ....

What were you doing? ....

What were you thinking? ....

Day ....

10																								
9																								
8																								
7																								
6																								
5																								
4																								
3																								
2																								
1																								
	1	2	3	4	5	6	7	8	9	10	11	12	1	2	3	4	5	6	7	8	9	10	11	12
						am						noon						pm						

At the end of the day, notice the period when you had the most cigarettes.

Where were you? ....

Who were you with? ....

What were you doing? ....

What were you thinking? ....

immediately after consumption. At least three problems may be encountered with this data. (1) Despite requests, clients may not complete the form regularly. Noncompliance can be anticipated by asking the client to complete the form at specified times such as at lunch and before going to bed, or by providing other environmental prompts. (2) Intoxication will often interfere with accurate recording, or the situation may make it difficult or embarrassing to write material down. This problem can be often avoided by asking clients to make a simple and unobtrusive count during the substance-use occasion, e.g. by passing a coin from one pocket to another each time they have a drink. Alternately, clients may monitor the products of usage, such as the number of bottles used, the number of remaining tablets or the number of cigarette butts. (3) Self-monitoring may initially be reactive, especially if recording is made before the substance use or if clients believe there are incentives attached to reduced consumption. Instructions to monitor consumption after the event and to keep it at normal levels may minimise this effect.

In view of the concerns that users may be inaccurate at reporting consumption (e.g. Midanik, 1982), other people are sometimes asked to make concurrent recordings or self-reports are tested against physiological measures. Each of these methods has limitations. Collateral informants also make recording errors, and may not be aware of some consumption. Many physiological measures are too expensive for regular application; others are only sensitive to very recent use or do not provide information on the amount consumed. Despite these problems, it is advisable to undertake checks on self-monitoring, since the expectation of these checks probably improves the accuracy of the monitoring data (Lowe, Windsor, Adams, Morris & Reese, 1986).

Cognitive assessment

Neuropsychological effects from chronic alcohol use include deficits in abstract thinking and in problem solving with novel or complex material (Chelune & Parker, 1981; Goldman, 1983). Since treatments often rely on these functions, individuals with cognitive deficits are likely to show poor outcomes unless the treatments are modified to reduce their cognitive demands (Becker & Jaffe, 1984; Gregson & Taylor, 1977; Sussman, Rychartik, Mueser, Glynn & Prue, 1986; Wilkinson & Sanchez-Craig, 1981).

When the client shows cognitive deficits, therapists are also advised to delay critical aspects of treatment for at least 21 days after withdrawal to capitalise on initial return of cognitive functioning (Wilkinson & Sanchez-Craig, 1981).

Behavioural measures

One common way of examining and training behaviours associated with drinking is to use a simulated bar setting. Within this setting, alcoholics have a greater speed of drinking, take large sips and order more unmixed drinks than people without alcohol problems (Sobell, Schaefer & Mills, 1972). Where the treatment goal is controlled drinking, these behaviours may be important targets for training. Since observations of drinkers in natural settings do not always show a differential response for alcoholics (Saunders & Richard, 1978), the behavioural assessment should preferably be within the person's usual drinking environment.

Medical assessment and physiological measures

Because of the severe medical consequences that often accompany substance abuse, it is advisable to refer the client for a thorough medical examination. Such a referral may be especially important when there is a risk of a severe withdrawal syndrome on cessation of the drug (e.g. after high levels of alcohol or barbiturates, or narcotics), or when there are other significant physical risks from the drug and the attendant lifestyle. Failure to initiate prompt medical treatment may prove life-threatening in some cases.

The usefulness of drug assays using blood, urine or breath samples will depend on the circumstances of the assessment and the speed with which the drug is metabolised. For example, blood-alcohol level (BAL) provides an indication of recent alcohol ingestion either through a direct analysis of a blood sample, or through breath analysis. A BAL of 0.01% is equivalent to 10 gms alcohol per 100 ml blood. Since a healthy person metabolises about 0.015% alcohol per hour, consumption of significant amounts of alcohol more than 12 hours before a testing may go undetected. Recent research on the use of adhesive skin patches that detect alcohol excreted in sweat (e.g. Phillips & McAloon, 1980) is a promising method of detecting alcohol use over a longer period. In the case of tobacco smoking, expired carbon monoxide provides information about smoking during the last few hours (Hughes, Frederiksen & Frazier, 1978), but detection over the last 12–24 hours requires measures such as saliva cotinine (Di Giusto & Eckard, 1986). Serum thiocyanate can detect smoking over around two weeks (Vogt, Selvin, Widdowson & Hulley, 1977).

Biochemical markers of chronic alcohol abuse include gamma-glutamyl transpeptidase, serum transaminases, erythrocyte mean cell colume, HDL-cholesterol and uric acid (Freedland, Frankel & Evenson, 1985; Papoz, Warnet, Pequignot, Eschwege, Claude & Schwartz, 1981; Rosalski & Rau, 1972; Whitfield, Hensley, Bryden & Gallagher, 1978). Combinations of biochemical tests discriminate heavy drinkers or alcoholics from lighter drinkers (e.g. Bernadt, Mumford, Taylor, Smith & Murray, 1982), but the tests have relatively poor sensitivity when they are used to discriminate heavy drinkers from an unselected community sample (e.g. Chick, Kreitman & Plant, 1981; Clark, Holder, Mullet & Whitehead, 1983; Skinner *et al.*, 1984). Sensitivity may be improved by combining biochemical and questionnaire measures (e.g. Kristenson & Trell, 1982).

Treatment of substance abuse

Selection of a treatment goal

Most treatment for substance dependence is orientated towards abstinence. Controversy still surrounds the adoption of a controlled drinking goal for people with alcohol problems, and particularly for individuals who Jellinek (1960) would have considered to be 'gamma' alcoholics (Heather & Robertson, 1983; Marlatt, 1983; Nathan & Skinstad, 1987). Current evidence suggests that a controlled drinking goal is best suited to people who: (a) request and have social support for it; (b) are less severely dependent on alcohol; (c) do not show severe physical or neuropsychological effects of alcohol abuse; and (d) are less than 40 years old and in regular employment (Heather & Robertson, 1983; Wilkinson & Sanchez-Craig, 1981). Provided these conditions are met, relapse from a controlled drinking goal does not appear to be greater than from abstinence (Miller & Baca, 1983).

For some individuals who refuse to alter their substance use, a treatment goal involving less hazardous use may be set. For example, narcotics users may be taught about needle sterilisation and educated about minimising the risks of accidental overdose. Heavy drinkers may be trained in maintaining adequate nutrition. To reduce the risk of AIDS transmission, clients may also be informed about safer sexual practices. If successful, these strategies may help prevent some of the more severe long-term health consequences without risking a tacit support of the person's abuse.

Treatment strategies

Reviews of cognitive/behavioural treatments for substance abuse are provided by Ashery (1985), Childress, McLellan & O'Brien (1985), Grabowski, Stitzer & Henningfield (1984), Miller (1980) and Stitzer, Bigelow & McCaul (1983). Components of a multi-faceted program may include:

1. *Development of motivation.* Motivational enhancement has already begun with an assessment interview that reviews some of the costs and benefits of the substance use. Motivation may be increased by altering environmental contingencies, for example, through training of the person's spouse (Sisson & Azrin, 1986). Attitude change and commitment may be enhanced by further education about the benefits of quitting and by involvement in persuading others and acting as models.

2. *Strategies to deal with problem stimuli.* In *stimulus-control*, situations that constitute especially high risk for relapse are identified and avoided (Carey & Maisto, 1985). Conversely, in *cue exposure* the person enters high-risk situations under supervision and is assisted to inhibit the substance-use response (Rankin, Hodgson & Stockwell, 1983).

3. *Contingency measurement.* Incentives may be used to encourage program attendance, assist the person to remain drug-free or to increase alternative behaviours (e.g. Bigelow, Stitzer, Griffiths & Liebson, 1981). To improve maintenance, naturally occurring incentives should be in place by the end of treatment.

4. *Development of inconsistent activities and coping skills.* Users are encouraged to increase activities that do not involve substance use and can be instituted at particular problem times. These changes are most likely to be maintained if they are rewarding or if they constitute a change in the person's social role: examples are finding a job, beginning new relationships and improving fitness (e.g. Azrin, 1976; Hunt & Azrin, 1973).

Specific skills to assist abstention may also be trained. For example, unassertive individuals may be trained to resist social pressure to use the substance (Van Hasselt, Hersen & Milliones, 1978). Attempts to deal with craving may involve diversion of attention, use of objectifying or externalising imagery, visualising the effects of relapse, or concentration on its time-limited nature (Marlatt & Gordon, 1985). Coping strategies may also be required to cope with sequelae of abstinence, such as weight gain after smoking cessation (Hall *et al.*, 1986).

5. *Problem-solving and decision-making skills.* Ideally, clients should be able to initiate contingency management, skill training or stimulus-control by themselves after treatment has concluded. For example, clients may be trained to anticipate high-risk situations, and generate strategies to reduce their frequency and deal with those that do occur (Chaney *et al.*, 1978).

6. *Aversive conditioning.* Aversive procedures can be used to reduce craving during abstinence, or to assist the development of controlled drinking skills (e.g. Lovibond & Caddy, 1970). Chemical stimuli have included emetine, which provokes vomiting (Voegtlin, 1940), and scoline, which induces paralysis (Thomson & Rathod, 1968). Antabuse (disulfiram) allows self-administered aversive trials for alcohol ingestion in the natural environment (Azrin, Sisson, Meyers & Godley, 1982), since unlike emetine or scoline, an aversive physiological reaction is only produced when alcohol is consumed. Problems with antabuse include medication compliance and the exclusion of many clients who show serious physical effects of alcohol abuse. Other procedures include production of motion sickness, electrical aversion and covert sensitisation (Miller, 1980).

When the substance itself has some unpleasant effects, treatment can emphasise these effects. Rapid smoking is a particularly successful example (Dahaner, 1977). Physical exclusions for this procedure have led to development of similar techniques such as rapid puffing, but these are typically not as powerful (Tiffany, Martin & Baker, 1986).

7. *Use of alternative forms of the substance.* Highly dependent clients are sometimes administered a similar substance, such as methadone for heroin users (Dole & Nyswander, 1965) or nicotine gum for tobacco smokers (Lam, Sze, Sacks & Chalmers, 1987). These

alternate preparations allow a graduated withdrawal from the substance, while immediately changing the topography of the substance use and allowing development of alternative behaviours (Dole & Nyswander, 1965). They are useful as adjunctive treatment (Killen, Maccoby & Taylor, 1984) but are less effective if they are applied without adequate advice or counselling (Kozlowski, 1984). In the case of methadone, there have been difficulties with estimation of dosage, illegal trafficking and clients who use it to simply deal with short-term problems in supply. The length and severity of withdrawal make it difficult to achieve a drug-free treatment outcome (Gossop, Bradley & Phillips, 1987; Reynolds & Magro, 1976).

8. *Additional skills for controlled use.* When clients have a goal of controlled use, they may need to develop skills in detecting the extent of their use and controlling the rate of ingestion. For example, subjects who are learning controlled drinking are given information on the amount of alcohol for particular blood-alcohol levels so that they can keep their consumption under those limits. This approach is favoured over one that trains drinkers to monitor internal sensations, since people with serious drinking problems are relatively poor at discriminating internal cues (Silverstein, Nathan & Taylor, 1974). When clients show problems in pacing their alcohol consumption, e.g. taking large or frequent sips and drinking spirits without mixers, they can be trained to develop alternative consumption behaviours (Sobell *et al.*, 1972).

9. *Bibliotherapy.* Cognitive-behavioural self-help manuals such as those by Miller & Munoz (1982) on drinking and Richmond & Webster (1985) on smoking are not only useful as adjuncts to other treatment, but may sometimes be legitimately used as the sole intervention without loss of effectiveness (Miller, Gribskov & Mortell, 1981; Miller & Taylor, 1980). This procedure may be particularly appropriate for less severe problems.

10. *Enhancement of social support.* When significant other people support a person's quit attempt, relapse risks are reduced (Mermelstein *et al.*, 1986). Mechanisms for this effect probably include assistance with stimulus-control, modelling of coping behaviour and maintenance of incentives for change. Positive relationships also help to avert interpersonal conflict and assist the person to deal with external stressors (Cohen & Wills, 1985). Initial attempts to foster great support from the person's family have not been very successful (Lichtenstein, Glasgow & Abrams, 1986), but encouraging interpersonal relationships within group

treatments does seem to benefit the participants (Hajek, Belcher & Stapelton, 1985).

One way to increase social support is for clients to join a self-help group such as Alcoholics Anonymous or Al-Anon (Edwards, Hensman, Hawker & Williamson, 1967; Leach, 1973). Available evidence suggests that the AA approach has a substantial impact, although its evaluation is usually confounded by self-selection and discontinuance (Miller & Hester, 1980). Its most potent active components probably include the prompts and strong social contingencies that are provided by other members, and the increases in relevant skills and self-efficacy that are given through advice and modelling by other members. Credibility of these components is enhanced by the fact that these individuals share the same problem and rapid delivery of assistance is provided through contacts between meetings. The movement also attempts to address the person's guilt about the problem by adopting a disease model that reduces personal responsibility. At the same time, it allows members to receive forgiveness and strength through its quasi-theistic philosophy and the corrective emotional experience that group meetings provide. Optimism is also enhanced through the adoption of daily goals, and attitude changes and commitment are maximised by voluntary involvement in persuading others. Many of these same features are provided by other groups with a substantial ex-user component. Residential community treatments of this kind offer a particularly high degree of contingency control, and extended group meetings intensify the power of social-influence processes. Clients who will accept the methods and philosophy of these groups may benefit from a referral.

Bibliography

Abramson, L. Y., Seligman, M. E. P. & Teasdale, J. D. (1978) 'Learned helplessness in humans: critique and reformulation.' *Journal of Abnormal Psychology*, *87*, 49–74

Ad Hoc Committee on the Classification of Headache (1962) 'Classification of headache.' *Journal of the American Medical Association*, *179*, 717–18

Adams, H. E., Feuerstein, M. & Fowler, J. L. (1980) 'Migraine headache: a review of parameters, etiology and intervention.' *Psychological Bulletin*, *87*, 217–37

Agras, W. S., Ferguson, J. M., Greaves, C., Qualls, B., Rand, C. S., Ruby, J., Stunkard, A. J., Taylor, C. B., Werne, J. & Wright, C. (1976) 'A clinical and research questionnaire for obese patients.' In B. J. Williams, S. Martin & J. P. Foreyt (eds), *Obesity: behavioral approaches to dietary management*. New York: Brunner/Mazel

Akiskal, H. S. & McKinney, W. T.; Jr. (1975) 'Overview of recent research in depression: integration of ten conceptual models into a comprehensive frame.' *Archives of General Psychiatry*, *32*, 285–305

Alden, L. & Safran, J. (1978) 'Irrational beliefs and assertive behavior.' *Cognitive Therapy and Research*, *2*, 357–64

Allison, W. M. & Jerrom, D. W. A. (1984) 'Glue sniffing: a pilot study of the cognitive effects of long-term use.' *The International Journal of the Addictions*, *19*, 453–58

Allon, N. (1982) 'The stigma of overweight in everyday life.' In B. B. Wolman (eds), *Psychological aspects of abesity: a handbook*. New York: Van Nostrand Reinhold, pp. 130–174

Alpert, R. & Haber, R. M. (1960) 'Anxiety in academic achievement situations.' *Journal of Abnormal and Social Psychology*, *61*, 207–15

American Psychiatric Association (1980) *Diagnostic and statistical manual of mental disorders*, 3rd edn, Washington, DC: American Psychiatric Association

American Psychiatric Association (1987) *Diagnostic and statistical manual of mental disorders*, 3rd edn (revised), Washington, DC: American Psychiatric Association

Anderson, B. J. & Wolfe, F. M. (1986) 'Chronic physical illness and behavior: Psychological issues.' *Journal of Consulting and Clinical Psychology*, *54*, 168–75

Andrasik, F. & Holroyd, K. A. (1980) 'Physiologic and self-report comparisons between tension headache sufferers and nonheadache controls.' *Journal of Behavioral Assessment*, *2*, 135–41

Annon, J. S. (1975) *The sexual pleasure inventory*. Honolulu: Enabling Systems Inc.

Archer, D. & Akert, R. M. (1977) 'Words and everything else: verbal and nonverbal cues in social interpretation.' *Journal of Personality and Social Psychology*, *35*, 443–9

Bibliography

Archibald, H. C. & Tuddenham, R. D. (1965) 'Persistent stress reaction after combat.' *Archives of General Psychiatry*, *12*, 475–81

Arena, J. G., Blanchard, E. B., Andrasik, F., Cotch, P. A. & Myers, P. E. (1983) 'Reliability of psychophysiological assessment.' *Behaviour Research and Therapy*, *21*, 447–60

Argyle, M. & Kendon, A. (1967) 'The experimental analysis of social performance.' In L. Berkowitz (ed), *Advances in experimental social psychology*, vol. 3, New York: Academic Press

Arkowitz, H. (1981) 'Assessment of social skills.' In M. Hersen & A. S. Bellack (eds), *Behavioural assessment: a practical handbook*, 2nd edn, New York: Pergamon Press

Ascher, L. M. & Efran, J. S. (1978) 'Use of paradoxical intention in a behavioral program for sleep onset insomnia.' *Journal of Consulting and Clinical Psychology*, *46*, 547–50

Ashery, R. S. (ed) (1985) *Progress in the development of cost-effective treatment for drug abusers.* NIDA Research Monograph 58, Rockville, MD: National Institute on Drug Abuse

Association of Sleep Disorders Centers (1979) *Sleep*, *2*, 1–137

Azrin, N. H. (1976) 'Improvements in the community-reinforcement approach to alcoholism.' *Behaviour Research and Therapy*, *14*, 339–48

Azrin, N. H., Sisson, R. W., Meyers, R. & Godley, M. (1982) 'Alcoholism treatment by disulfiram and community reinforcement therapy.' *Journal of Behavior Therapy and Experimental Psychiatry*, *13*, 105–12

Babor, T. F. Cooney, N. L. & Laverman, R. J. (1987) 'The dependence syndrome concept as a psychological theory of relapse behavior: an empirical evaluation of alcohol and opiate addicts.' *British Journal of Addiction*, *82*, 393–405

Bakal, D. A. (1982) *The psychobiology of chronic headache.* New York: Springer

——— & Kaganov, J. A. (1977) 'Muscle contraction and migraine headache: a psychophysiological comparison.' *Headache*, *17*, 208

Baker, A. L. & Wilson, P. H. (1985) 'Cognitive-behavior therapy for depression: the effects of booster sessions on relapse.' *Behavior Therapy*, *16*, 335–44

Baker, B. L., Cohen, D. C. & Saunders, J. T. (1973) 'Self-directed desensitization for acrophobia.' *Behaviour Research and Therapy*, *11*, 78–89

Bandura, A. (1977a) *Social learning theory.* Englewood Cliffs, N.J.: Prentice-Hall

——— (1977b) 'Self-efficacy: toward a unifying theory of behavioral change.' *Psychological Review*, *84*, 191–215

——— (1982) 'Self-efficacy mechanism in human agency.' *American Psychologist*, *37*, 122–47

——— (1986) *Social foundations of thought and action: a social cognitive theory.* Englewood Cliffs, NJ: Prentice-Hall

———, Blanchard, E. B. & Ritter, B. (1969) 'Relative efficacy of desensitization and modeling approaches for inducing behavioral, affective, and attitudinal changes.' *Journal of Personality and Social Psychology*, *13*, 173–99

———, Jeffrey, R. W. & Wright, C. L. (1974) 'Efficacy of participant modeling as a function of response induction aids.' *Journal of Abnormal Psychology*, *83*, 56–64

———, Reese, L. & Adams, N. E. (1982) 'Microanalysis of action and fear arousal as a function of differential levels of perceived self-efficacy.' *Journal of Personality and Social Psychology*, *43*, 5–21

——— & Rosenthal, T. L. (1966) 'Vicarious classical conditioning as a function of arousal level.' *Journal of Personality and Social Psychology*, *3*, 54–62

Barlow, D. H. (ed) (1981) *Behavioral assessment of adult disorders*. New York: Guilford

——— (ed) (1985) *Clinical handbook of psychological disorders: a step-by-step treatment manual*. New York: Guilford

———, Abel, G. G. Blanchard, E. B., Bristow, A. R. & Young, L. D. (1977) 'A heterosocial skills behavior checklist for males.' *Behavior Therapy*, *8*, 229–39

Beck, A. T. & Emery, G. (1979) *Cognitive therapy of anxiety and phobic disorders*. Philadelphia: Center for Cognitive Therapy

———, Rush, A. J., Shaw, B. F. & Emery, G. (1979) *Cognitive therapy of depression*. New York: Guilford

———, Ward, C. H., Mendelson, M., Mock, J. & Erbaugh, J. (1961) 'An inventory for measuring depression.' *Archives of General Psychiatry*, *4*, 561–71

Becker, J. T. & Jaffe, J. H. (1984) 'Impaired memory for treatment-related information in inpatient men alcoholics.' *Journal of Studies on Alcohol*, *45*, 440–52

Becker, R. E. & Heimberg, R. G. (1985) 'Cognitive-behavioral treatments for depression: a review of controlled clinical research.' In A. Dean (ed), *Depression in multidisciplinary perspective*, New York: Brunner/Mazel

Bellack, A. S. (1979) 'A critical appraisal of strategies for assessing social skill.' *Behavioral Assessment*, *1*, 157–76

——— & Hersen, M. (1978) 'Chronic psychiatric patients: social skills training.' In M. Hersen & A. S. Bellack (eds), *Behavioral therapy in the psychiatric setting*, Baltimore: Williams and Wilkins

———, Hersen, M. & Turner, S. M. (1978) 'Role play tests for assessing social skills: are they valid?' *Behavior Therapy*, *9*, 448–61

Bentler, P. M. (1967) 'Heterosexual behaviour assessment. I. Males.' *Behaviour Research and Therapy*, *5*, 90

——— (1968) 'Heterosexual behaviour assessment. II. Females'. *Behaviour Research and Therapy*, *6*, 27–30

Bernadt, M. W., Mumford, J., Taylor, C., Smith, B. & Murray, R. M. (1982) 'Comparison of questionnaire and laboratory tests in the detection of excessive drinking and alcoholism.' *Lancet*, *1*, 325–8

Bernstein, D. A. & Allen, G. T. (1969) 'Fear survey schedule (II): normative data and factor analyses based upon a large college sample.' *Behaviour Research and Therapy*, *7*, 403–7

——— & Borkovec, T. D. (1973) *Progressive relaxation training: a manual for the helping professions*. Champaign, IL: Research Press

Best, J. A. & Hakstian, A. R. (1978) 'A situation-specific model for smoking behavior.' *Addictive Behaviors*, *3*, 79–92

Beumont, P., Al-Alami, M. & Touyz, S. (1987) 'Relevance of standard measurement of undernutrition to the diagnosis of anorexia nervosa: use of Quetelet's body mass index (BMI).' *International Journal of Eating Disorders* (in press)

Bibb, J. L. & Chambless, D. L. (1986) 'Alcohol use and abuse among diagnosed alcoholics.' *Behaviour Research and Therapy, 24*, 49–58

Bigelow, G., Stitzer, M. L. Griffiths, R. R. & Liebson, I. A. (1981) 'Contingency management approaches to drug self-administration and drug abuse: efficacy and limitations.' *Addictive Behaviors, 6*, 241–52

Birrell, P. C. (1983) 'Behavioral, subjective, and electroencephalographic indices of sleep onset latency and duration.' *Journal of Behavioral Assessment, 5*, 179–90

Bjorntorp, P., Carlgren, G., Isaksson, B., Krotkiewski, M., Larsson, B. & Sjostrom, L. (1975) 'Effect of an energy-reduced dietary regimen in relation to adipose tissue cellularity in obese women.' *American Journal of Clinical Nutrition, 28*, 445–52

——— & Sjostrom, L. (1971) 'Number and size of adipose fat cells in relation to metabolism in human obesity.' *Metabolism, 20*, 703–13

Blanchard, E. B., Ahles, T. A. & Shaw, E. R. (1979) 'Behavioral treatment of headaches.' In M. Hersen, R. M. Eisler & P. M. Miller (eds), *Progress in behavior modification*, vol. 8, New York: Academic Press

——— & Andrasik, F. (1982) 'Psychological assessment and treatment of headache: recent developments and emerging issues.' *Journal of Consulting and Clinical Psychology, 50*, 859–79

——— & ——— (1985) *Management of chronic headaches: a psychological approach*. New York: Pergamon Press

———, ———, Ahles, T. A., Teders, S. J. & O'Keefe, D. M. (1980) 'Migraine and tension headache: a meta-analytic review.' *Behavior Therapy, 11*, 613–31

———, ———, Arena, J. G., Neff, D. F., Saunders, N. L., Jurish, S. E., Teders, S. J. & Rodichok, L. (1983) 'Psychophysiological responses as predictors of response to behavioral treatment of headache.' *Behavior Therapy, 14*, 357–74

———, ———, Neff, D. F., Jurish, S. E. & O'Keefe, D. M. (1981) 'Social validation of the headache diary.' *Behavior Therapy, 12*, 711–15

———, ———, ———, Arena, J. G., Ahles, T. A., Jurish, S. E., Pallmeyer, T. P., Saunders, N. L., Teders, S. J., Barron, K. D. & Rodichok, L. D. (1982) 'Biofeedback and relaxation training with three kinds of headache: treatment effects and their prediction.' *Journal of Consulting and Clinical Psychology, 50*, 562–75

Blane, H. T. & Leonard, K. E. (eds) (1987) *Psychological theories of drinking and alcoholism*. New York: Guilford

Bootzin, R. R. & Engle-Friedman, M. (1981) 'The assessment of insomnia.' *Behavioral Assessment, 3*, 107–26

——— & Nicassio, P. M. (1978) 'Behavioral treatments for insomnia.' In M. Hersen, R. M. Eisler & P. M. Miller (eds), *Progress in behavior modification*, vol. 6, New York: Academic Press

Borkovec, T. D. (1982) 'Insomnia.' *Journal of Consulting and Clinical Psychology, 50*, 880–95

Bowlby, J. (1969) *Attachment and loss. Vol. 1: Attachment*. London: Hogarth Press

Boyle, G. J. (1985) 'Self-report measures of depression: some psychometric considerations.' *British Journal of Clinical Psychology*, *24*, 45–9

Brasted, W. S. & Callahan, E. J. (1984) 'A behavioral analysis of the grief process.' *Behavior Therapy*, *15*, 529–43

Braude, M. C. & Chao, H. M. (eds) (1986) *Genetic and biological markers in drug abuse and alcoholism*. NIDA Monograph 66. Rockville, MD: National Institute on Drug Abuse

Braun, P. R. & Reynolds, D. J. (1969) 'A factor analysis of a 100-item fear survey inventory.' *Behaviour Research and Therapy*, *7*, 399–402

Bray, G. A. (1976) *The obese patient*. Philadelphia: Saunders

Brewin, C. R. (1985) 'Depression and causal attributions: what is their relation?' *Psychological Bulletin*, *98*, 297–309

Brown, G. W. & Harris, T. O. (1978) *Social origins of depression*. London: Tavistock Press

Brown, S. A., Goldman, M. S., Inn, A. & Anderson, L. R. (1982) 'Expectations of reinforcement from alcohol: their domain and relation to drinking patterns.' *Journal of Consulting and Clinical Psychology*, *48*, 419–26

Brownell, K. D. (1981) 'Assessment of eating disorders.' In D. H. Barlow *Behavioral assessment of adult disorders*, New York: Guilford

——— (1982) 'Obesity: understanding and treating a serious, prevalent and refractory disorder.' *Journal of Consulting and Clinical Psychology*, *50*, 820–40

——— (1984) 'The addictive disorders.' In G. T. Wilson, C. M. Franks, K. D. Brownell & P. C. Kendall (eds), *Annual review of behavior therapy: theory & practice*, New York: Guilford

———, Marlatt, G. A., Lichtenstein, E. & Wilson, G. T. (1986) 'Understanding and preventing relapse.' *American Psychologist*, *41*, 765–82

Bryant, P. M. & Trower, P. (1974) 'Social difficulty in a student sample.' *British Journal of Educational Psychology*, *44*, 13–21

Bryant, B. M., Trower, P., Yardley, K., Urbieta, H. & Letemendia, F. (1976) 'A survey of social inadequacy among psychiatric outpatients.' *Psychological Medicine*, *6*, 101–12

Budzynski, T. H., Stoyva, J. M. Adler, C. S. & Mullaney, D. J. (1973) 'EMG biofeedback and tension headache: a controlled outcome study.' *Psychosomatic Medicine*, *35*, 484–96

Buglass, D., Clarke, J., Henderson, A. S., Kreitman, N. & Presley, A. S. (1977) 'A study of agoraphobic housewives.' *Psychological Medicine*, *7*, 73–86

Burns, E. L. & Thorpe, G. L. (1977) 'Fears and clinical phobias: epidemiological aspects and the national survey of agoraphobics.' *Journal of International Medical Research*, *5*, 132–9

Butler, L. & Meichenbaum, D. (1981) 'The assessment of interpersonal problem solving skills.' In P. C. Kendall & S. D. Hollon (eds), *Assessment strategies for cognitive behavioral interventions*, New York: Academic Press

Callner, D. A. & Ross, S. M. (1976) 'The reliability and validity of three measures of assertion in a drug addict population.' *Behavior Therapy*, *7*, 659–67

Carey, K. B. & Maisto, S. A. (1985) 'A review of the use of self-control techniques in the treatment of alcohol abuse.' *Cognitive Therapy and Research*, *9*, 235–51

Carroll, B. J., Feinberg, M., Smouse, P. E., Rawson, S. G. & Greden, J. F. (1981) 'The Carroll rating scale for depression: I. development, reliability and validation.' *British Journal of Psychiatry*, *138*, 194–200

Cervone, D. (1985) 'Randomization tests to determine significance levels for microanalytic congruences between self-efficacy and behavior.' *Cognitive Therapy and Research*, *9*, 357–65

Chambless, D. L., Caputo, G. C., Jasin, S. E., Gracely, E. J. & Williams, C. (1985) 'The mobility inventory for agoraphobia.' *Behaviour Research and Therapy*, *23*, 35–44

Chaney, E. F., O'Leary, M. R. & Marlatt, G. A. (1978) 'Skill training with alcoholics.' *Journal of Consulting and Clinical Psychology*, *46*, 1092–1104

Chase, J. L., Salzberg, H. C. & Palotai, A. M. (1984) 'Controlled drinking revisited: a review.' In M. Hersen, R. M. Eisler & P. M. Miller (eds), *Progress in Behavior Modification*. vol. 18, New York: Academic Press

Chelune, G. J. & Parker, J. B. (1981) 'Neuropsychological deficits associated with chronic alcohol abuse.' *Clinical Psychology Review*, *1*, 181–95

Chick, J. (1980) 'Is there a unidimensional alcohol dependence syndrome?' *British Journal of Addiction*, *75*, 265–80

——, Kreitman, N. & Plant, M. (1981) 'Mean cell volume and gamma-glutamyl-transpeptidase as markers of drinking in working men.' *Lancet*, *I*, 1249–51

Childress, A. R., McLellan, A. T. & O'Brien, C. P. (1985) 'Behavioural therapies for substance abuse.' *The International Journal of the Addictions*, *20*, 947–69

Christakis, G. (1975) 'The prevalence of adult obesity.' In G. A. Bray (ed), *Obesity in perspective*, Department of Health, Education and Welfare (NIH) 75–708, Washington, DC

Christiansen, B. A., Goldman, M. S. & Inn, A. (1982) 'Development of alcohol-related expectancies in adolescents: separating pharmacological from social-learning influences of reinforcement from alcohol: their domain and relation to drinking patterns.' *Journal of Consulting and Clinical Psychology*, *50*, 336–44

Cimminero, A. R., Calhoun, K. S. & Adams, H. E. (1977) *Handbook of behavioral assessment*. New York: Wiley

Clark, P., Holder, R., Mullet, M. & Whitehead, T. P. (1983) 'Sensitivity and specificity of laboratory tests for alcohol abuse.' *Alcohol and Alcoholism*, *18*, 261–9

Cobb, J., McDonald, R., Marks, I. & Stern, R. (1980) 'Marital versus exposure therapy: psychological treatments of co-existing marital and phobic-obsessive problems.' *Behaviour Analysis and Modification*, *4*, 3–16

Cohen, S. & Wills, T. A. (1985) 'Stress, social support, and the buffering hypothesis.' *Psychological Bulletin*, *98*, 310–57

Colvin, R. H. & Olson, S. B. (1983) 'A descriptive analysis of men and women who have lost significant weight and are highly successful at maintaining the loss.' *Addictive Behaviors*, *8*, 287–95

Condiotte, M. M. & Lichtenstein, E. (1981) 'Self-efficacy and relapse in smoking cessation programs.' *Journal of Consulting and Clinical Psychology*, *49*, 648–58

Connolly, J., Hallam, R. S. & Marks, I. M. (1976) 'Selective association of fainting with blood-illness-injury fear.' *Behavior Therapy*, *7*, 8–13

Cooney, N. L., Meyer, R. E., Kaplan, R. F. & Baker, L. H. (1986) 'A validation study of four scales measuring severity of alcohol dependence.' *British Journal of Addiction*, *81*, 223–9

Coyne, J. C. (1976) 'Depression and the response of others.' *Journal of Abnormal Psychology*, *85*, 186–93

——— & Gotlib, I. H. (1983) 'The role of cognition in depression: a critical appraisal.' *Psychological Bulletin*, *94*, 472–505

——— & ——— (1986) 'Studying the role of cognition in depression: well-trodden paths and cul-de-sacs.' *Cognitive Therapy and Research*, *10*, 695–705

Craighead, W. E., Kazdin, A. E. & Mahoney, M. J. (1981) *Behavior modification: issues, principles, and application*. Dallas: Houghton-Mifflin

Crowe, R. R., Noyes, R., Pauls, D. L. & Slymen, D. (1983) 'A family study of panic disorder.' *Archives of General Psychiatry*, *40*, 1065–69

Curran, J. P. (1977) 'Skills training as an approach to the treatment of heterosexual social anxiety: a review.' *Psychological Bulletin*, *84*, 140–57

———, Corriveau, D. P., Monti, P. M. & Hagerman, S. (1980) 'Social skill and social anxiety: self-report measurement in a psychiatric population.' *Behavior Modification*, *4*, 493–512

Curry, S., Marlatt, G. A. & Gordon, J. R. (1987) 'Abstinence violation effect: validation of an attributional construct with smoking cessation.' *Journal of Consulting and Clinical Psychology*, *55*, 145–9

Cutrona, C. E. (1982) 'Nonpsychotic postpartum depression: a review of recent research.' *Clinical Psychology Review*, *2*, 487–503

Dahaner, B. G. (1977) 'Research on rapid smoking: interim summary and recommendations.' *Addictive Behaviors*, *2*, 155–66

Delprato, D. J. (1980) 'Hereditary determinants of fears and phobias: a critical review.' *Behavior Therapy*, *11*, 79–103

Depue, R. A. (1979) *The psychobiology of depressive disorders: implications for the effects of stress*. New York: Academic Press

——— & Monroe, S. M. (1978) 'The unipolar-bipolar distinction in the depressive disorders.' *Psychological Bulletin*, *85*, 10001–29

Derogatis, L. R., Meyer, J. D. & Dupkin, C. N. (1976) 'Discrimination of organic vs. psychogenic impotence with the DSFI.' *Journal of Sex and Marital Therapy*, *2*, 229–40

DeSilva, P., Rachman, S. & Seligman, M. E. P. (1977) 'Prepared phobias and obsessions: therapeutic outcome.' *Behaviour Research and Therapy*, *15*, 65–77

Diamond, S. (1983) 'Depression and headache.' *Headache*, *13*, 122

DiClimente, C. C. (1981) 'Self-efficacy and smoking cessation maintenance: a preliminary report.' *Cognitive Therapy and Research*, *5*, 175–87

Di Giusto, E. & Eckhard, I. (1986) 'Some properties of saliva cotinine measurements in indicating exposure to tobacco smoking.' *American Journal of Public Health*, *76*, 1–2

DiNardo, P. A., O'Brien, G. T., Barlow, D. H., Waddell, M. T. & Blanchard, E. B. (1983) 'Reliability of DSM-III anxiety disorder categories using a new structured interview.' *Archives of General Psychiatry*, *40*, 1070–4

Dittrich, J., Houts, A. C. & Lichstein, K. L. (1983) 'Panic disorder: assessment and treatment.' *Clinical Psychology Review*, *3*, 215–25

Dobson, K. S. & Breiter, H. J. (1983) 'Cognitive assessment of depression: reliability and validity of three measures.' *Journal of Abnormal Psychology*, *92*, 107–9

Dole, V. P. & Nyswander, M. A. (1965) 'Medical treatment for diacetyl morphine (heroin) addiction.' *Journal of the American Medical Association*, *193*, 645–56

Donovan, D. M. & Marlatt, G. A. (1980) 'Assessment of expectancies and behaviors associated with alcohol consumption: a cognitive-behavioral approach.' *Journal of Studies on Alcohol*, *41*, 1153–85

Durnin, J. V., Armstrong, W. H. & Womersley, J. (1973) 'An experimental study on the variability of measurement of skinfold thickness by three observers on 23 young women and 27 young men.' *Human Biology*, *45*, 281–92

Eastman, C. (1984) *Drink and drinking problems*. New York: Longman

Edwards, G., Hensman, C., Hawker, A. & Williamson, V. (1967) 'Alcoholics Anonymous: the anatomy of a self-help group.' *Social Psychiatry*, *1*, 195–204

Eisler, R. M., Hersen, M., Miller, P. M. & Blanchard, E. B. (1975) 'Situational determinants of assertive behaviour.' *Journal of Consulting and Clinical Psychology*, *43*, 330–40

Emmelkamp, P. M. G. (1979) 'The behavioral study of phobias.' In M. Hersen, R. M. Eisler & P. M. Miller (eds), *Progress in behavior modification*, vol. 8, New York: Academic Press

Endicott, J., Cohen, J., Nee, J., Fleiss, J. & Sarantakos, S. (1981) 'Hamilton depression rating scales: extracted from regular and change versions of the schedule for affective disorders and schizophrenia.' *Archives of General Psychiatry*, *38*, 98–103

——— & Spitzer, R. L. (1978) 'A diagnostic interview. The schedule for affective disorders and schizophrenia.' *Archives of General Psychiatry*, *35*, 837–44

Erdlen, R., McLellan, A. T., La Porte, D. J., *et al.* (1978) *Instruction manual for the administration of the addiction severity index*. Philadelphia: Veterans Administration Press

Etringer, B. D., Cash, T. F. & Rimm, D. C. (1982) 'Behavioral, affective, and cognitive effects of participant modeling and an equally credible placebo.' *Behavior Therapy*, *13*, 476–85

Evenson, R. C. (1986) 'The Missouri alcoholism severity scale: relationship with type of alcohol consumption.' *Journal of Studies on Alcohol*, *47*, 381–2

———, Holland, R. A. & Cho, D. W. (1979) 'A scale for measuring the severity of alcoholism and evaluating its treatment.' *Journal of Studies on Alcohol*, *40*, 1077–81

Ewing, J. A. (1984) 'Detecting alcoholism: the CAGE questionnaire.' *Journal of the American Medical Association*, *252*, 1905–7

Eysenck, H. J. & Eysenck, S. B. G. (1964) *Manual of the Eysenck personality inventory*. London: University of London Press

——— & ——— (1975) *Manual of the Eysenck personality questionnaire*. Sevenoaks, Kent: Hodder and Stoughton

Fagerstrom, K. O. (1982) 'A comparison of psychological and pharmacological treatments in smoking cessation.' *Journal of Behavioral Medicine*, *5*, 343–51

Fairbank, J. A. & Brown, T. A. (1987) 'Current behavioral approaches to the treatment of post-traumatic stress disorder.' *The Behavior Therapist*, *10*, 57–64

Fennell, M. J. V. & Campbell, E. A. (1984) 'The cognitions questionnaire: specific thinking errors in depression.' *British Journal of Clinical Psychology*, *23*, 81–91

Fischer, S. C. & Turner, R. M. (1978) 'Standardization of the fear survey schedule.' *Journal of Behavior Therapy and Experimental Psychiatry*, *9*, 129–33

Foa, E. B., Steketee, G. & Young, M. C. (1984) 'Agoraphobia: phenomenological aspects, associated characteristics, and theoretical considerations.' *Clinical Psychology Review*, *4*, 431–57

Foch, T. T. & McClearn, G. E. (1980) 'Genetics, body weight and obesity.' In A. J. Stunkard (ed), *Obesity*, Philadelphia: W. B. Saunders, pp. 48–71

Foreyt, J. P. & Kondo, A. T. (1984) 'Advances in behavioral treatment of obesity.' In M. Hersen, R. M. Eisler & P. M. Miller (eds), *Progress in behavior modification*, vol. 16. New York: Academic Press

Foster, A. L. (1977) 'The sexual compatibility test.' *Journal of Consulting and Clinical Psychology*, *45*, 332–3

Frankel, B. L., Coursey, R., Buchbinder, R. & Snyder, F. (1976) 'Recorded and reported sleep in chronic primary insomnia.' *Archives of General Psychiatry*, *33*, 615–23

Franklin, J. A. (1984) 'Agoraphobia: Its nature, development, maintenance, and treatment.' Unpublished Ph.D. thesis, University of New South Wales, Sydney

Franzini, L. R. & Grimes, W. B. (1976) 'Skinfold measures as the criterion of change in weight control studies.' *Behavior Therapy*, *7*, 256–9

Freedland, K. E., Frankel, M. T. & Evenson, R. C. (1985) 'Biochemical diagnosis of alcoholism in men psychiatric patients.' *Journal of Studies on Alcohol*, *46*, 103–6

Freedman, R. R. & Papsdorf, J. D. (1976) 'Biofeedback and progressive relaxation treatment of sleep-onset insomnia: a controlled all-night investigation.' *Biofeedback and Self Regulation*, *1*, 253–71

——— & Sattler, H. L. (1982) 'Physiological and psychological factors in sleep onset insomnia.' *Journal of Abnormal Psychology*, *91*, 380–9

Freund, K. & Blanchard, R. (1981) 'Assessment of sexual dysfunction and deviation.' In M. Hersen & A. S. Bellack (eds), *Behavioral assessment: a practical handbook*, New York: Pergamon Press

Frisancho, A. R. (1981) 'New norms of upper limb fat and muscle areas for assessment of nutritional status.' *American Journal of Clinical Nutrition*, *34*, 2540–5
Fuchs, C. Z. & Rehm, L. P. (1977) 'A self-control behavior therapy program for depression.' *Journal of Consulting and Clinical Psychology*, *45*, 206–15
Gaardner, K. R. & Montgomery, P. S. (1977) *Clinical biofeedback: a procedural manual*. Baltimore: Williams & Wilkins
Gambrill, E. D. & Richey, C. A. (1975) 'An assertion inventory for use in assessment and research.' *Behavior Therapy*, *6*, 550–61
Garrow, J. (1974) *Energy balance and obesity in man*. New York: Elsevier
Garssen, B., Van Veenendaal, W. & Bloemink, R. (1983) 'Agoraphobia and the hyperventilation syndrome.' *Behaviour Research and Therapy*, *21*, 643–9
Gawin, F. H. & Kleber, H. D. (1986) 'Abstinence symptomatology and psychiatric diagnosis in cocaine abusers: clinical observations.' *Archives of General Psychiatry*, *43*, 107–13
Geer, J. H. (1965) 'The development of a scale to measure fear.' *Behaviour Research and Therapy*, *3*, 45–53
Glaister, B. (1982) 'Muscle relaxation training for fear reduction of patients with psychological problems: a review of controlled studies.' *Behaviour Research and Therapy*, *20*, 493–504
Godding, P. R. & Glasgow, R. E. (1985) 'Self-efficacy and outcome expectations as predictors of controlled smoking status.' *Cognitive Therapy and Research*, *9*, 583–90
Goldfried, M. R. & Sprafkin, J. N. (1976) 'Behavioral personality assessment.' In J. T. Spence, R. C. Carson & J. W. Thibaut (eds), *Behavioral approaches to therapy*. Morristown, N.J.: General Learning Press
Goldman, M. S. (1983) 'Cognitive impairment in chronic alcoholics: some cause for optimism.' *American Psychologist*, *38*, 1045–54
Goldstein, A. J. & Chambless, D. L. (1978) 'A reanalysis of agoraphobia.' *Behavior Therapy*, *9*, 47–59
Goldstein, A. P. (1973) *Structured learning therapy: towards a psychotherapy for the poor*. New York: Academic Press
———, Sherman, M., Gershaw, N. J., Sprafkin, B. & Glick, B. (1978) 'Training aggressive adolescents in prosocial behavior.' *Journal of Youth and Adolescence*, 773–93
Gormally, J., Sipps, G., Raphael, R., Edwin, D. & Varvil-Wald, D. (1981) 'The relationship between maladaptive cognitions and social anxiety.' *Journal of Consulting and Clinical Psychology*, *49*, 300–1
Gossop, M., Bradley, B. & Phillips, G. T. (1987) 'An investigation of withdrawal symptoms shown by opiate addicts during and subsequent to a 21-day in-patient methadone detoxification procedure.' *Addictive Behaviors*, *12*, 1–6
Grabowski, J. (ed) (1984) *Cocaine: pharmacology, effects, and treatment of abuse*. NIDA Research Monograph 50. Rockville, MD: National Institute on Drug Abuse
———, Stitzer, M. L. & Henningfield, J. E. (1984) *Behavioral intervention techniques in drug abuse treatment*. NIDA Research Monograph 46.

Rockville, MD: National Institute on Drug Abuse

Grande, F. (1975) 'Assessment of body fat in man.' In G. A. Bray (ed), *Obesity in perspective*, Dept. of Health, Education and Welfare, NIH 75–708, Washington, DC

Grattan, W. G., Wilson, P. H. & Franklin, J. (1987) *Respiratory retraining, cognitive modification and relaxation training versus supportive psychotherapy in the preparation of agoraphobics for in-vivo exposure*. Manuscript in submission

Gregson, R. A. M. & Stacey, B. G. (1982) 'Self-reported alcohol consumption: a real psychophysical problem.' *Psychological Reports*, *50*, 1027–33

——— & Taylor, G. M. (1977) 'Prediction of relapse in men alcoholics.' *Journal Studies on Alcohol*, *38*, 1749–60

Hajek, P., Belcher, M. & Stapelton, J. (1985) 'Enhancing the impact of groups: an evaluation of two group formats for smokers.' *British Journal of Clinical Psychology*, *24*, 289–294

Hall, S. M. (1984) 'The abstinence phobias: links between substance abuse and anxiety.' *The International Journal of the Addictions*, *19*, 613–31

———, Ginsberg, D. & Jones, R. T. (1986) 'Smoking cessation and weight gain.' *Journal of Consulting and Clinical Psychology*, *54*, 342–6

———, Tunstall, C., Rugg, D., Jones, R. T. & Benowitz, N. (1985) 'Nicotine gum and behavioral treatment in smoking cessation.' *Journal of Consulting and Clinical Psychology*, *53*, 256–8

Halmi, K. A., Stunkard, A. J. & Mason, E. E. (1980) 'Emotional responses to weight reduction by three methods: gastric bypass, jejunoileal bypass and diet.' *American Journal of Clinical Nutrition*, *33*, 446–51

Hamilton, M. (1959) 'The assessment of anxiety states by rating.' *British Journal of Medical Psychology*, *32*, 50–9

——— (1960) 'A rating scale for depression.' *Journal of Neurology, Neurosurgery and Psychiatry*, *23*, 56–62

Hargie, O., Saunders, C. & Dickson, D. (1981). *Social skills in interpersonal communication*. London: Croom Helm

Harper, M. & Roth, M. (1962) 'Temporal lobe epilepsy and the phobic anxiety-depersonalization syndrome. Part I: a comparative study.' *Comprehensive Psychiatry*, *3*, 129–51

Harris, M. B. & Hallbauer, E. S. (1973) 'Self-directed weight control through eating and exercise.' *Behaviour Research and Therapy*, *11*, 523–9

Harrison, R. H. (1975) 'Psychological testing and headache: a review.' *Headache*, *15*, 177

Hauri, P. J. (1981) 'Treating psychophysiologic insomnia with biofeedback.' *Archives of General Psychiatry*, *38*, 752–8

Hauri, P. J., Percy, L., Hellekson, C., Hartmann, E. & Russ, D. (1982) 'The treatment of psychophysiologic insomnia with biofeedback: a replication study.' *Biofeedback and Self-Regulation*, *7*, 223–35

Hawton, K., Catalan, J., Martin, P. & Fagg, J. (1986) 'Long term outcome of sex therapy.' *Behaviour Research and Therapy*, *24*, 665–75

Haynes, S. N., Adams, West, S., Kamens, L. & Safranek, R. (1982) 'The stimulus control paradigm in sleep-onset insomnia: a multimethod assessment.' *Journal of Psychosomatic Research*, *26*, 333–9

———, ———, A. E. & Franzen, M. (1981) 'The effects of pre-sleep stress on sleep-onset insomnia.' *Journal of Abnormal Psychology*, *90*, 601–6
———, Follingstad, D. R. & McGowan, W. T. (1974) 'Insomnia, sleep patterns and anxiety level.' *Journal of Psychosomatic Research*, *18*, 69–74
Healey, E. S., Kales, A., Monroe, L. J., Bixler, E. O., Chamberlain, K. & Soldatos, C. R. (1981) 'Onset of insomnia: role of life-stress events.' *Psychosomatic Medicine*, *43*, 439–51
Heather, N. & Robertson, I. (1983) *Controlled drinking*. London: Methuen
Heiman, J., LoPiccolo, L. & LoPiccolo, J. (1976) *Becoming orgasmic: a sexual growth programme for women*. New Jersey: Prentice-Hall
Hersen, M. (1973) 'Self-assessment of fear.' *Behavior Therapy*, *4*, 241–57
——— & Bellack, A. S. (1976) 'Social skills training for chronic psychiatric patients. Rationale, research findings and future directions.' *Comprehensive Psychiatry*, *17*, 559–80
——— & ——— (1981) *Behavioral assessment: a practical handbook*. New York: Pergamon Press
———, ———, Himmelhoch, J. M. & Thase, M. E. (1984) 'Effects of social skill training, amitriptyline, and psychotherapy in unipolar depressed women.' *Behavior Therapy*, *15*, 21–40
Hesselbrock, M., Babor, T. F., Hesselbrock, V., Meyer, R. E. & Workman, K. (1983) ' "Never believe an alcoholic"? On the validity of self-report measures of alcohol dependence and related constructs.' *The International Journal of the Addictions*, *18*, 593–609
———, Meyer, R. E. & Keener, J. J. (1985) 'Psychopathology in hospitalized alcoholics.' *Archives of General Psychiatry*, *42*, 1050–5
Hillenberg, J. B. & Collins, F. L. (1982) 'A procedural analysis and review of relaxation training research.' *Behaviour Research and Therapy*, *20*, 251–60
Hodgson, R. J., Stockwell, T., Rankin, H. & Edwards, G. (1978) 'Alcohol dependence: the concept, its utility and measurement.' *British Journal of Addiction*, *73*, 339–42
Hollon, S. D. & Kendall, P. C. (1980) 'Cognitive self-statements in depression: development of an automatic thoughts questionnaire.' *Cognitive Therapy and Research*, *4*, 383–95
Holroyd, K. A. & Andrasik, F. (1978) 'Coping and the self-control of chronic tension headache.' *Journal of Consulting and Clinical Psychology*, *45*, 1036–45
———, ——— & Westbrook, T. (1977) 'Cognitive control of tension headache.' *Cognitive Therapy and Research*, *1*, 121–33
Hoon, E. F., Hoon, P. W. & Wincze, J. P. (1976) 'An inventory for the measurement of female arousibility: the SAI.' *Archives of Sexual Behavior*, *5*, 291–301
Hopkins, J., Marcus, M. & Campbell, S. B. (1984) 'Postpartum depression: a critical review.' *Psychological Bulletin*, *95*, 498–515
Horn, J. L., Wanberg, K. W. & Foster, F. M. (1974) *The Alcohol Use Inventory — AUI*. Denver, Colo: Center for Alcohol-Abuse Research and Evaluation
Howarth, E. & Schokman-Gates, K. (1981) 'Self-report multiple mood instruments.' *British Journal of Psychology*, *72*, 421–41
Hughes, J. R., Frederiksen, L. W. & Frazier, M. (1978) 'A carbon

monoxide analyzer for measurement of smoking behavior.' *Behavior Therapy*, *9*, 293–6

——— & Hatsukami, D. (1986) 'Signs and symptoms of tobacco withdrawal.' *Archives of General Psychiatry*, *43*, 289–94

Hull, J. (1981) 'A self-awareness model of the causes and effects of alcohol consumption.' *Journal of Abnormal Psychology*, *90*, 586–600

Hunt, G. M. & Azrin, N. H. (1973) 'The community-reinforcement approach to alcoholism.' *Behaviour Research and Therapy*, *11*, 91–104

Hurt, R. D., Morse, R. M. & Swenson, W. M. (1980) 'Diagnosis of alcoholism with a self-administered alcoholism screening test: results with 1,002 consecutive patients receiving general examinations.' *Mayo Clinic Proceedings*, *55*, 365–70

Institute of Medicine (1982) *Marihuana and health*. Washington, DC: National Academy Press

Istvan, J. & Matarazzo, J. D. (1984) 'Tobacco, alcohol, and caffeine use: A review of their interrelationships.' *Psychological Bulletin*, *95*, 301–26

Jacob, R. G., Turner, S. N., Szekely, B. C. & Eidelman, B. H. (1983) 'Predicting outcome of relaxation therapy in headaches: the role of depression.' *Behavior Therapy*, *14*, 457–65

Jacobson, G. R. (1984) 'Detection, assessment and diagnosis of alcoholism: current techniques.' In M. Galanter (ed), *Recent developments in alcoholism*, New York: Plenum

James, J. E. & Crosbie, J. (1987) 'Somatic and psychological health implications of heavy caffeine use.' *British Journal of Addiction*, *82*, 503–9

Jehu, D. (1979) *Sexual dysfunction: a behavioural approach to causation, assessment and treatment*. Chichester: Wiley

Jellinek, E. M. (1960) *The disease concept of alcoholism*. New Brunswick, NJ: Hillhouse Press

Kales, A. & Kales, J. (1984) *Evaluation and treatment of insomnia*. New York: Oxford University Press

Kaloupek, D. G. & Levis, D. J. (1983) 'Issues in the assessment of fear: response concordance and prediction of avoidance behavior.' *Journal of Behavioral Assessment*, *5*, 239–60

Kanfer, F. H. & Saslow, G. (1969) 'Behavioral diagnosis.' In C. M. Franks (ed), *Behavior therapy: appraisal and status*, New York: McGraw-Hill

Kanner, A. D., Coyne, J. C., Schaefer, C. A. & Lazarus, R. S. (1981) 'Comparison of two modes of stress management: daily hassles and uplifts versus major life events.' *Journal of Behavioral Medicine*, *4*, 1–39

Kaplan, H. (1974) *The new sex therapy: active treatment of sexual dysfunction*. New York: Brunner/Mazel.

———, Pokorney, A., Kanes, T. & Lively, G. (1974) 'Screening tests and self-identification in the detection of alcoholism.' *Journal of Health and Social Behavior*, *15*, 51–60

Kavanagh, D. J. & Wilson, P. H. (1987, in submission) *Prediction of outcome with cognitive therapy for depression*.

———, Knight, D. A. & Ponzio, V. (1986) 'In vivo practice for needle phobia: report on two cases.' *Behaviour Change*, *3*, 63–9

Kazarian, S. S., Howe, M. G. & Csapo, K. G. (1979) 'Development of the sleep behavior self-rating scale.' *Behavior Therapy*, *10*, 412–17

Kearney, B. G., Wilson, P. H. & Haralambous, G. (1987) 'Stress appraisal and personality characteristics of headache patients: comparisons with tinnitus and normal control groups.' *Behaviour Change*, *4*, 25–32

Keesey, R. E. (1980) 'A set-point analysis of the regulation of body weight.' In A. J. Stunkard (ed), *Obesity*, Philadelphia: Saunders

Keller, M. B., Shapiro, R. W., Lavori, P. W. & Wolfe, N. (1982) 'Relapse in major depressive disorder: analysis of the life table.' *Archives of General Psychiatry*, *39*, 911–15

Kelley, J. E. & Lichstein, K. L. (1980) 'A sleep assessment device.' *Behavioral Assessment*, *2*, 135–46

Kendall, P. C. & Hollon, S. D. (eds) (1979) *Cognitive-behavioral interventions: theory, research, and procedures*. New York: Academic Press

———, ———, Beck, A. T., Hammen, C. L. & Ingram, R. E. (1987) 'Issues and recommendations regarding use of the Beck depression inventory.' *Cognitive Therapy and Research*, *11*, 289–99

Kendell, R. E. (1976) 'The classification of depressions: a review of contemporary confusion.' *British Journal of Psychiatry*, *129*, 15–28

Keys, A. (1975) 'Overweight and the risk of heart attack and sudden death.' In G. A. Bray (ed), *Obesity in Perspective*, Department of Health, Education and Welfare (NIH) 75–708, Washington, DC

Killen, J. D., Maccoby, N. & Taylor, C. B. (1984) 'Nicotine gum and self-regulation training in smoking relapse prevention.' *Behavior Therapy*, *15*, 234–48

King, N. J. (1980) 'The therapeutic utility of abbreviated progressive relaxation: a critical review with implications for clinical practice.' In M. Hersen, R. M. Eisler & P. M. Miller (eds), *Progress in behavior modification*, vol. 10, New York: Academic Press

Klein, D. F. (1981) 'Anxiety reconceptualized.' In D. F. Klein & J. Rabkin (eds), *Anxiety: new research and changing concepts*, New York: Raven Press, pp. 235–263

Knesevich, J. W., Biggs, J. T., Clayton, P. J. & Ziegler, V. E. (1977) 'Validity of the Hamilton rating scale for depression.' *British Journal of Psychiatry*, *131*, 49–52

Knight, R. G., Waal-Manning, J. and Spears, G. F. (1983) 'Some norms and reliability data for the state–trait anxiety inventory and the Zung self-rating depression scale.' *British Journal of Clinical Psychiatry*, *22*, 245–9

Kornblith, A. B. (1981) 'Multiple drug use involving nonopiate, nonalcoholic substances. II. Physical damage, long-term effects and treatment approaches and success.' *The International Journal of the Addictions*, *16*, 527–40

Kotin, J., Wilbert, D. E., Verburg, D. & Soldinger, S. M. (1976) 'Thioridazine and sexual dysfunction.' *American Journal of Psychiatry*, *133*, 82–5

Kozlowski, L. T. (1984) 'Pharmacological approaches to smoking modification.' In J. D. Matarazzo, Sharlene M. Weiss, J. A. Herd, N. E. Miller & Stephen M. Weiss (eds), *Behavioural health: a handbook of health enhancement and disease prevention*, New York: Wiley

Krantz, S. & Hammen, C. (1979) 'Assessment of cognitive bias in depression.' *Journal of Abnormal Psychology*, *88*, 611–19

Krasnegor, N. A. (ed) (1979) *Cigarette smoking as a dependence process*. NIDA Research Monograph 23. Rockville, MD: National Institute on Drug Abuse

Kristenson, H. & Trell, E. (1982) 'Indicators of alcohol consumption: comparisons between a questionnaire (Mm–MAST), interviews and serum gamma-glutamyl transferase (GGT), in a health survey of middle-aged males.' *British Journal of Addiction*, *77*, 297–304

Krosnick, A. & Podolsky, S. (1981) 'Diabetes and sexual dysfunction: restoring normal ability.' *Geriatrics*, *36*, 92–100

Krug, S. E., Scheier, I. H. & Cattell, R. B. (1976) *Handbook for the IPAT anxiety scale*, 2nd edn, Champaign, IL: Institute for Personality and Ability Testing

Lacey, J. I. & Lacey, B. B. (1968) 'Verification and extension of the principle of automatic response stereotypy.' *American Journal of Psychology*, *71*, 50–73

Lacks, P. (1987) *Behavioral treatment for persistent insomnia*. New York: Pergamon

———, Bertelson, A. D., Gans, L. & Kunkel, J. (1983) 'The effectiveness of three behavioral treatments for different degrees of sleep onset insomnia.' *Behavior Therapy*, *14*, 593–605

Ladd, G. W. & Mize, J. (1983) 'A cognitive-social learning model of social-skill training.' *Psychological Review*, *90*, 127–57

Lader, M. H. & Mathews, A. M. (1970) 'Physiological changes during spontaneous panic attacks.' *Journal of Psychosomatic Research*, *14*, 377–82

Lam, W., Sze, P. C., Sacks, H. S. & Chalmers, T. C. (1987) 'Meta-analysis of randomized controlled trials of nicotine chewing-gum.' *The Lancet*, 4 July, 27–9

Lang, P. J. (1968) 'Fear reduction and fear behavior: problems in treating a construct.' In J. Shlien (ed), *Research in psychotherapy*, vol. 3, Washington, DC: American Psychological Association

——— (1971) 'The application of psychophysiological methods to the study of psychotherapy and behavior change.' In A. E. Bergin & S. L. Garfield (eds), *Handbook of psychotherapy and behavior change: an empirical analysis*, New York: Wiley

——— (1977) 'Physiological assessment of anxiety and fear.' In J. D. Cone & R. P. Hawkins (eds), *Behavioral assessment: new directions in clinical psychology*, New York: Brunner/Mazel, pp. 178–95

——— & Lazovik, A. D. (1963) 'Experimental desensitization of a phobia.' *Journal of Abnormal and Social Psychology*, *66*, 519–25

———, Melamed, B. G. & Hart, J. (1970) 'A psychophysiological analysis of fear modification using an automated desensitization procedure.' *Journal of Abnormal Psychology*, *76*, 220–34

Larcombe, N. A. & Wilson, P. H. (1984) 'An evaluation of cognitive-behaviour therapy for depression in patients with multiple sclerosis.' *British Journal of Psychiatry*, *145*, 366–71

Last, C. G. (1984) 'Cognitive treatment of phobia.' In M. Hersen, R. M. Eisler & P. M. Miller (eds), *Progress in behavior modification*, vol.

16, New York: Academic Press

Leach, B. (1973) 'Does Alcoholics Anonymous really work?' In P .G. Bourne & R. Fox (eds), *Alcoholism: progress in research and treatment*, New York: Academic Press

Le Bow, M. (1984) *Child obesity: a new frontier of behavior therapy*. New York: Springer

Lehrer, P. M. & Woolfolk, R. L. (1982) 'Self-report assessment of anxiety: somatic, cognitive, and behavioral modalities.' *Behavioral Assessment*, *4*, 167–77

Leitenberg, H., Agras, W. S., Butz, R. & Wincze, J. (1971) 'Relationship between heart rate and behavioral change during the treatment of phobias.' *Journal of Abnormal Psychology*, *78*, 59–68

Lew, E. A. & Garfinkel, L. (1979) 'Variations in mortality by weight among 750,000 men and women.' *Journal of Chronic Diseases*, *32*, 563–76

Lewinsohn, P. M. (1975) 'The behavioral study and treatment of depression.' In M. Hersen, R. M. Eisler & P. M. Miller (eds), *Progress in behavior modification*, vol. 1, New York: Academic Press

———, Antonuccio, D., Steinmetz, J. & Teri, L. (1984) *The coping with depression course*, Eugene, Ore: Castalia

———, Hoberman, H., Teri, L. & Hautzinger, M. (1985) 'An integrative theory of depression.' In S. Reiss & R. R. Bootzin (eds), *Theoretical issues in behavior therapy*, New York: Academic Press

———, Mischell, W., Chaplin, W. & Barton, R. (1980) 'Social competence and depression: the role of illusory self-perception.' *Journal of Abnormal Psychology*, *89*, 203–12

———, Marmelstein, R. M., Alexander, C. & MacPhillamy, D. J. (1985) 'The unpleasant events schedule: a scale for the measurement of aversive events.' *Journal of Clinical Psychology*, *41*, 483–98

———, Youngren, M. A. & Grosscup, S. J. (1979) 'Reinforcement and depression.' In R. A. Depue (ed), *The psychobiology of depressive disorders: implications for the effects of stress*, New York: Academic Press

Ley, P. (1980) 'The psychology of obesity: its causes, consequences and control.' In S. Rachman (ed), *Contributions to medical psychology*, vol. 2, Oxford: Pergamon Press

——— (1984) 'Some tests of the hypothesis that obesity is a defence against depression.' *Behaviour Research and Therapy*, *22*, 197–9

Liberman, R. P., King, L. W., De Risi, W. J. & McCann, M. (1975) *Personal effectiveness: guiding people to assert themselves and improve their social skills*. Champaign, IL: Research Press

Libet, J. M. & Lewinsohn, P. M. (1973) 'Concept of social skill with special reference to the behavior of depressed persons.' *Journal of Consulting and Clinical Psychology*, *40*, 304–12

Lichtenstein, E., Glasgow, R. E. & Abrams, D. B. (1986) 'Social support in smoking cessation: in search of effective interventions.' *Behavior Therapy*, *17*, 607–19

Lichstein, K. L., Nickel, R., Hoelscher, T. J. & Kelley, J. E. (1982) 'Clinical validation of a sleep assessment device.' *Behaviour Research and Therapy*, *20*, 292–7

——— & Rosenthal, T. L. (1980) 'Insomniacs' perceptions of cognitive versus somatic determinants of sleep disturbance.' *Journal of Abnormal*

Psychology, *89*, 105–7

Lief, H. I. & Reed, D. M. (1972) *Sexual knowledge and attitude test. (SKAT).* Pennsylvania: Center for the Study of Sex Education in Medicine, University of Pennsylvania

Linden, W. (1981) 'Exposure treatments for focal phobias: a review.' *Archives of General Psychiatry*, *38*, 769–75

——— & Wright, J. (1980) 'Programming generalization through social skills training in the natural environment.' *Behaviour Analysis and Modification*, *4*, 239–51

Linton, P. H. & Estock, M. D. (1977) 'The anxiety phobic depersonalization syndrome: role of the cognitive-perceptual style.' *Diseases of the Nervous System*, *38*, 138–41

Locke, H. J. & Wallace, K. M. (1959) 'Short marital adjustment and prediction tests: Their reliability and validity.' *Marriage and Family Living*, 251–5

LoPiccolo, J. & LoPiccolo, L. (1978) *Handbook of sex therapy.* New York: Plenum

——— & Steger, J. C. (1974) 'The sexual interaction inventory: a new instrument for assessment of sexual dysfunction.' *Archives of Sexual Behaviour*, *3*, 585–95

——— & Stock, W. E. (1986) 'Treatment of sexual dysfunction.' *Journal of Consulting and Clinical Psychology*, *54*, 158–67

Lovibond, S. H. (1979) *Objective methods of sleep recording in the study and management of insomnia.* Paper delivered at the Conference of the Australian Behaviour Modification Association, Adelaide

——— & Caddy, G. R. (1970) 'Discriminated aversive control in the moderation of alcoholics' drinking behaviour.' *Behaviour Therapy*, *1*, 437–44

Lowe, J. B., Windsor, R. A., Adams, B., Morris, J. & Reese, Y. (1986). 'Use of a bogus pipeline method to increase accuracy of self-reported alcohol consumption among pregnant women.' *Journal of Studies on Alcohol*, *47*, 173–5

Lowe, M. R. (1982) 'Validity of the positive behavior subscale of the social performance survey schedule in a psychiatric population.' *Psychological Reports*, *50*, 83–7

——— (1985) 'Psychometric evaluation of the social performance survey schedule.' *Behavior Modification*, *9*, 193–210

——— & Cautela, J. R. (1978) 'A self-report measure of social skill.' *Behavior Therapy*, *9*, 535–44

——— & Fisher, E. B. (1983) 'Emotional reactivity, emotional eating and obesity: a naturalistic study.' *Journal of Behavioral Medicine*, *6*, 135–49

Lubin, B. (1965) 'Adjective checklists for measurement of depression.' *Archives of General Psychiatry*, *12*, 57–62

Ludwig, A. M. & Wikler, A. (1984) ' "Craving" and relapse to drink.' *Quarterly Journal of Studies on Alcohol*, *35*, 108–30

Lutwak, L. & Coulston, A. (1975) 'Activity and obesity.' In G. A. Bray (ed), *Obesity in perspective*, Department of Health, Education and Welfare (NIH), 75–708, Washington, DC

MacAndrew, C. (1965) 'The differentiation of male alcoholic outpatients from nonalcoholic psychiatric outpatients by means of the MMPI.' *Quarterly Journal of Studies on Alcohol*, *26*, 238–46

MacPhillamy, D. & Lewinsohn, P. M. (1982) 'The pleasant events schedule: studies on reliability, validity, and scale intercorrelation.' *Journal of Consulting and Clinical Psychology, 50*, 363–80

MacRae, J. R., Scoles, M. T. & Siegel, S. (1987) 'The contribution of Pavlovian conditioning to drug tolerance and dependence.' *British Journal of Addiction, 82*, 371–80

Madden, J. S. (1979) *A guide to alcohol and drug dependence*. Bristol: John Wright & Sons

Mahoney, M. J. (1974) *Cognition and behavior modification*. Cambridge, Mass.: Ballinger

Margolin, G. & Jacobson, N. S. (1981) 'Assessment of marital dysfunction.' In M. Hersen and A. S. Bellack (eds), *Behavioral assessment: a practical handbook*, New York: Pergamon

Marks, I. M. (1970) 'Agoraphobic syndrome.' *Archives of General Psychiatry, 23*, 538–53

——— & Gelder, M. G. (1966) 'Different ages of onset in varieties of phobia.' *American Journal of Psychiatry, 123*, 218–21

——— & Herst, E. R. (1970) 'A survey of 1,200 agoraphobics in Britain.' *Social Psychiatry, 5*, 16–24

——— & Mathews, A. M. (1979) 'Brief standard self-rating for phobic patients.' *Behaviour Research and Therapy, 17*, 263–7

Marlatt, G. A. (1983) 'The controlled drinking controversy: a commentary.' *American Psychologist, 38*, 1097–1110

——— & Gordon, J. (eds) (1985) *Relapse prevention: maintenance strategies in the treatment of addictive behaviors*. New York: Guilford

Martin, P. R. & Matthews, A. M. (1978) 'Tension headaches: psychophysiological investigation and treatment.' *Journal of Psychosomatic Research, 22*, 389–99

Marzillier, J. S., Lambert, C. & Kellet, J. (1976) 'A controlled evaluation of systematic densensitization and social skills training for socially inadequate psychiatric patients.' *Behaviour Research and Therapy, 14*, 225–38

Masters, W. & Johnson, V. (1966) *Human sexual response*. Boston: Little, Brown and Co.

——— & ——— (1970) *Human sexual inadequacy*. Boston: Little, Brown and Co.

Mathews, A. M. Gelder, M. G. & Johnston, D. W. (1981) *Agoraphobia: nature and treatment*. London: Tavistock

Mathews, A., Teasdale, J., Munby, M., Johnston, D. & Shaw, P. (1977) 'A home-based treatment program for agoraphobia.' *Behaviour Therapy, 8*, 915–24

Mayer, J. E. & Filstead, W. J. (1979) 'The adolescent alcohol involvement scale: an instrument for measuring adolescents' use and misuse of alcohol.' *Journal of Studies on Alcohol, 40*, 291–300

Mayfield, D., Mcleod, G. & Hall, P. (1974) 'The CAGE questionnaire: validation of a new alcoholism screening instrument.' *American Journal of Psychiatry, 131*, 1121–3

McFall, R. M. (1982) 'A review and reformulation of the concept of social skills.' *Behavioral Assessment, 4*, 1–33

McGlynn, F. D., Mealiea, W. L. & Landau, D. L. (1981) 'The current

status of systematic densensitization.' *Clinical Psychology Review, 1,* 149–79
McGovern, K. B., Stewart, R. D. & LoPiccolo, J. (1975) 'Secondary orgasmic dysfunction I. Analysis and strategies for treatment.' *Archives of Sexual Behavior, 4,* 265–75
McIntyre, K. O., Lichtenstein, E. & Mermelstein, R. J. (1983) 'Self-efficacy and relapse in smoking cessation: a replication and extension.' *Journal of Consulting and Clinical Psychology, 51,* 632–3
McKnight, D. L., Nelson, R. O., Hayes, S. C. & Jarrett, R. B. (1984) 'Importance of treating individually assessed response classes in the amelioration of depression.' *Behavior Therapy, 14,* 315–35
McLean, P. D. & Hakstian, A. R. (1979) 'Clinical depression: comparative efficacy of outpatient treatments.' *Journal of Consulting and Clinical Psychology, 47,* 818–36
McLellan, A. T., Luborsky, L., Cacciola, J., Griffith, J., Evans, F., Barr, H. & O'Brien, C. (1985) 'New data from the addiction severity index: reliability and validity in three centers.' *The Journal of Nervous and Mental Disease, 173,* 412–23
———, Luborsky, L. Woody, G. E. & O'Brien, C. P. (1980) 'An improved diagnostic evaluation instrument for substance abuse patients: the addiction severity index.' *The Journal of Nervous and Mental Disease, 168,* 26–33
McNeal, E. T. & Cimbolic, P. (1986) 'Antidepressants and biochemical theories of depression.' *Psychological Bulletin, 99,* 361–74
Meichenbaum, D. H. (1977) *Cognitive-behavior modification: an integrative approach.* New York: Plenum Press
Mellinger, G. D., Balter, M. B. & Uhlenhuth, E. H. (1985) 'Insomnia and its treatment: prevalence and correlates.' *Archives of General Psychiatry, 42,* 225–32
Mellor, C. S. (1970) 'Nomogram for calculating mass of alcohol in different beverages.' *British Medical Journal,* 703.
Mendel, J. G. & Klein, D. F. (1969) 'Anxiety attacks with subsequent agoraphobia.' *Comprehensive Psychiatry, 10,* 190–5
Mermelstein, R., Cohen, S., Lichtenstein, E., Baer, J. S. & Kamark, T. (1986) 'Social support and smoking cessation maintenance.' *Journal of Consulting and Clinical Psychology, 54,* 447–53
Midanik, L. (1982) 'The validity of self-reported alcohol consumption and alcohol problems: a literature review.' *British Journal of Addiction, 77,* 357–82
Milby, J. B., Gurwitch, R. H., Wiebe, D. J., Ling, W., McLellan, T. & Woody, G. E. (1986) 'Prevalence and diagnostic reliability of methadone maintenance detoxification fear.' *American Journal of Psychiatry, 143,* 739–43
Miller, L. S. & Funabiki, D. S. (1984) 'Predictive validity of the social performance survey schedule for component interpersonal behaviors.' *Behavioral Assessment,* 33–44
Miller, W. R. (ed) (1980) *The addictive behaviours: treatment of alcoholism, drug abuse, smoking and obesity.* Oxford: Pergamon Press
——— & Baca, L. M. (1983) 'Two-year follow-up of bibliotherapy and therapist-directed controlled drinking training for problem drinkers.'

Behavior Therapy, *14*, 441–8
———, Gribskov, C. J. & Mortell, R. L. (1981) 'Effectiveness of a self-control manual for problem drinkers and without therapist contact.' *International Journal of the Addictions*, *16*, 1247–54
——— & Hester, R. K. (1980) 'Treating the problem drinker: modern approaches.' In W. R. Miller (ed), *The addictive behaviours: treatment of alcoholism, drug abuse and obesity*. Oxford: Pergamon Press, pp. 11–141
——— & Munoz, R. F. (1982) *How to control your drinking*, revised edn, Albuquerque, NM: University of New Mexico Press
——— & Seligman, M. E. P. (1975) 'Depression and learned helplessness in man.' *Journal of Abnormal Psychology*, *84*, 228–38
——— & Taylor, C. A. (1980) 'Relative effectiveness of bibliotherapy, individual and group self-control training in the treatment of problem drinkers.' *Addictive Behaviors*, *5*, 13–24
Mischel, W. (1968) *Personality and assessment*. New York: Wiley
Mitchell, K. R. (1979) 'Behavioral treatment of pre-sleep tension and intrusive cognitions in patients with severe pre-dormital insomnia.' *Journal of Behavioral Medicine*, *2*, 57–69
——— & White, R. G. (1977) 'Self-management of severe pre-dormital insomnia.' *Journal of Behavior and Experimental Psychiatry*, *8*, 57–63
Moberg, D. P. (1983) 'Identifying adolescents with alcohol problems: a field test of the adolescent involvement scale.' *Journal of Studies on Alcohol*, *44*, 701–21
Monroe, L. (1967) 'Psychological and physiological differences between good and poor sleepers.' *Journal of Consulting and Clinical Psychology*, *72*, 255–64
Morrison, R. L. & Bellack, A. (1981) 'The role of social perception in social skills.' *Behavior Therapy*, *12*, 69–79
Morse, R. M. & Hurt, R. D. (1979) 'Screening for alcoholism.' *Journal of the American Medical Association*, *242*, 2688–90
Moss, R. A. (1987, in press) 'New approaches in the assessment and treatment of chronic headaches.' *Journal of Pain Management Practice*
———, Garrett, J. & Chiodo, J. F. (1982) 'Temporomandibular joint dysfunction and myofascial pain dysfunction syndromes: parameters, etiology, and treatment.' *Psychological Bulletin*, *92*, 331–45
———, McClure, J. T., Jackson, M. C. & Lombardo, T. (1987) 'The influence of sleep duration on headache pain and frontalis EMG.' *Journal of Oral Rehabilitation*, *14*, 331–5
Mowrer, O. H. (1947) 'On the dual nature of learning: a reinterpretation of "conditioning" and "problem solving".' *Harvard Educational Review*, *17*, 102–48
Murphy, G. E., Simons, A. D., Wetzel, R. D. & Lustman, P. J. (1984) 'Cognitive therapy and pharmacotherapy: singly and together in the treatment of depression.' *Archives of General Psychiatry*, *41*, 33–41
Myers, J. K., Weissman, M. M., Tischler, G. L., Holzer, C. E., Leaf, P. J., Orvaschel, H., Anthony, J. C., Boyd, J. H., Burke, J. D., Kramer, M. & Stoltzman, R. (1984) 'Six-month prevalence of psychiatric disorders in three communities.' *Archives of General Psychiatry*, *41*, 959–67
Nathan, P. E. & Skinstad, A.-H. (1987) 'Outcome of treatment for

alcohol problems: current methods, problems and results.' *Journal of Consulting and Clinical Psychology*, *55*, 332–40

Nay, W. R. (1979) *Multimethod clinical assessment*. New York: Gardner Press

Nezu, A. M. (1986) 'Efficacy of a social problem solving therapy approach for unipolar depression.' *Journal of Consulting and Clinical Psychology*, *54*, 196–202

Nicassio, P. M., Mendlowitz, D. R., Fussell, J. J. & Petras, L. (1985) 'The phenomenology of the pre-sleep state: the development of the pre-sleep arousal scale.' *Behaviour Research and Therapy*, *23*, 263–71

Ohman, A., Eriksson, A. & Olofsson, C. (1975) 'One-trial learning and superior resistance to extinction of autonomic responses conditioned to potentially phobic stimuli.' *Journal of Comparative and Physiological Psychology*, *88*, 619–27

Oliver, J. M. & Baumgart, E. P. (1985) 'The dysfunctional attitude scale: psychometric properties and relation to depression in an unselected adult population.' *Cognitive Therapy and Research*, *9*, 161–7

Ollendick, T. M. (1979) 'Fear reduction techniques with children.' In M. Herson, R. M. Eisler & P. M. Miller (eds), *Progress in behavior modification*, vol 8, New York: Academic Press

Orford, J. (1985) *Excessive appetites: a psychological view of addiction*. Chichester: John Wiley

Ornstein, P. (1976) 'The Alcadd test as a predictor of post-hospital drinking behavior.' *Psychological Reports*, *43*, 611–17

Öst, L. G., Jerremalm, A. & Jansson, L. (1984) 'Individual response patterns and the effects of different behavioral methods in the treatment of agoraphobia.' *Behaviour Research and Therapy*, *22*, 697–707

Osterhouse, R. A. (1972) 'Desensitization and study-skills training as treatment for two types of test-anxious students.' *Journal of Counselling Psychology*, *19*, 301–7.

Papoz, L., Warnet, J-M., Pequignot, G., Eschwege, E., Claude, J. R. & Schwartz, B. (1981) 'Alcohol consumption in a healthy population: relationship to glutamyltransferase activity and mean corpuscular volume.' *Journal of the American Medical Association*, *245*, 1748–51

Paul, G. L. (1966) *Insight vs. desensitization in psychotherapy*. Stanford, CA: Stanford University Press

Paykel, E. S., Myers, J. K., Dienelt, M. N., Klerman, G. L., Lindenthal, J. J. & Pepper, M. P. (1969) 'Life events and depression: a controlled study.' *Archives of General Psychiatry*, *21*, 753–60

Perera, K. M. H., Tulley, M. & Jenner, F. A. (1987) 'The use of benzodiazepines among drug addicts.' *British Journal of Addiction*, *82*, 511–15

Philips, C. (1977) 'Psychological analysis of tension headache.' In S. J. Rachman (ed), *Contributions to medical psychology*, vol 1, Oxford: Pergamon Press

——— (1978) 'Tension headache: theoretical problems.' *Behaviour Research and Therapy*, *16*, 249–61

Phillips, M. & McAloon, M. H. (1980) 'A sweat-patch test for alcohol consumption: evaluation in continuous and episodic drinkers.' *Alcoholism: Clinical and Experimental Research*, *4*, 391–5

Platt, J. J. & Spivak, G. (1975) *Manual for the Means-Ends Problem-Solving*

Procedures (MEPS). Philadelphia: Department of Mental Health Services

Pokorney, A. D., Miller, B. A. & Kaplan, H. B. (1972) 'The brief MAST: a shortened version of the Michigan alcoholism screening test.' *American Journal of Psychiatry*, *129*, 342–5

Polich, J. N., Armour, D. J. & Braiker, H. B. (1980) 'Patterns of alcoholism over four years.' *Journal of Studies on Alcohol*, *41*, 397–416

Power, M. J. & Champion, L. A. (1986) 'Cognitive approaches to depression: a theoretical critique.' *British Journal of Clinical Psychology*, *25*, 201–12

Powers, P. S. (1980) *Obesity: the regulation of weight*. Baltimore: Williams & Williams

Pozniak-Patewicz, E. (1976) '"Cephalic" spasm of head and neck muscles.' *Headache*, *15*, 261–6

Preng, K. W. & Clopton, J. R. (1986) 'The MacAndrew scale: clinical application and theoretical issues.' *Journal of Studies on Alcohol*, *47*, 228–36

Prochaska, J. O. & DiClimente, C. C. (1983) 'Stage processes of self-change in smoking: toward an integrative model of change.' *Journal of Consulting and Clinical Psychology*, *51*, 390–5

Rachman, S. J. (1976) 'The passing of the two-stage theory of fear and avoidance: fresh possibilities.' *Behaviour Research and Therapy*, *14*, 125–34

—— (1977) 'The conditioning theory of fear acquistion: a critical examination.' *Behaviour Research and Therapy*, *15*, 375–87

—— & Hodgson, R. J. (1974) 'Synchrony and dysynchrony in fear and avoidance.' *Behaviour Research and Therapy*, *12*, 311–18

Radloff, L. S. (1977) 'The CES-D scale: a self-report depression scale for research in the general population.' *Applied Psychological Measurement*, *1*, 385–401

Raistrick, D., Dunbar, G. & Davidson, R. (1983) 'Development of a questionnaire to measure alcohol dependence.' *British Journal of Addiction*, *78*, 89–95

Rankin, H. J., Hodgson, R. J. & Stockwell, T. R. (1983) 'Cue exposure and response prevention with alcoholics: a controlled trial.' *Behaviour Research and Therapy*, *21*, 435–46

——, Stockwell, T. & Hodgson, R. (1982) 'Cues for drinking and degrees of alcohol dependence.' *British Journal of Addiction*, *77*, 287–96

Rapee, R., Mattick, R. & Murrell, E. (1986, May) 'Cognitive mediation in the affective component of spontaneous panic attacks.' Paper presented at the Annual Conference of Australian Behaviour Modification Association, Sydney

Raskin, A. & Crook, T. H. (1976) 'The endogenous-neurotic distinction as a predictor of response to antidepressant drugs.' *Psychological Medicine*, *6*, 59–70

Rathjen, D. P. (1980) 'An overview of social competence.' In D. P. Rathjen & J. P. Foreyt (eds), *Social competence: interventions for children and adults*, New York: Pergamon Press

Rehm, L. P. (1977) A self-control model of depression. *Behavior Therapy*, *8*, 787–804

—— (1981) 'Assessment of depression.' In M. Hersen & A. S. Bellack (eds), *Behavioral assessment: a practical handbook*, New York: Pergamon Press

Reynolds, I. & Magro, D. (1976) 'The use of methadone as a treatment tool for opiate addicts: a two-year follow-up study.' *The Medical Journal of Australia*, *9*, 560–2

Rice, K M. & Blanchard, E. B. (1982) 'Biofeedback in the treatment of anxiety disorders.' *Clinical Psychology Review*, *2*, 557–77

Richardson, F. C. & Tasto, D. L. (1976) 'Development and factor analysis of a social anxiety inventory.' *Behavior Therapy*, *7*, 453–62

Richmond, R. & Webster, I. (1985) *Become a non-smoker*. Sydney: Butterworths

Rimm, D. C. & Lefebvre, R. C. (1981) 'Phobic disorders.' In S. M. Turner, K. S. Calhoun & H. E. Adams (eds), *Handbook of clinical behaviour therapy*, New York: Wiley, pp. 12–40

Rist, F. & Watzl, H. (1983) 'Self-assessment of relapse risk and assertiveness in relation to treatment outcome of female alcoholics.' *Addictive Behaviours*, *8*, 121–7

Robinson, C. H. & Annon, J. S. (1975) *The Heterosexual Behavior Inventory*. Honolulu: Enabling Systems Inc.

Rogers, T., Mahoney, M. J. & Mahoney, B. K. (1980) 'Clinical assessment of obesity: an empirical evaluation of diverse techniques.' *Behavioral Assessment*, *2*, 161–81

Rosalski, S. B. & Rau, D. (1972) 'Serum gamma-glutamyl transpeptidase activity in alcoholism.' *Clinical Chimica Acta*, *39*, 41–7

Rosekind, M. R., Coates, T. J. & Thoresen, C. E. (1978) 'Telephone transmission of polysomnographic data from subjects' homes.' *Journal of Nervous and Mental Disease*, *166*, 438–41

Rosenbaum, M. (1980) 'A schedule for assessing self-control behaviors: preliminary findings.' *Behavior Therapy*, *11*, 109–21

Rosenthal, R., Hall, J. A., DiMatteo, M., Rogers, P. & Archer, D. (1979) *Sensitivity to nonverbal communications: the PONS test*. Baltimore: Johns Hopkins University Press

Roth, D., Bielski, R., Jones, M., Parker, W. & Osborn, G. (1982) 'A comparison of self-control therapy and combined self-control therapy and antidepressant medication in the treatment of depression.' *Behavior Therapy*, *13*, 133–44

Ruff, G. A., Moss, R. A. & Lombardo, T. W. (1986) 'Common migraine: a review and proposal for a non-vascular aetiology.' *Journal of Oral Rehabilitation*, *13*, 499–508

Rush, A. J. (ed) (1982) *Short-term psychotherapies for depression*. New York: Guilford

——, Giles, D. E., Schlesser, M. A., Fulton, C. L., Weissenburger, J. & Burns, C. (1986) 'The inventory for depressive symptomatology (IDS): preliminary findings.' *Psychiatry Research*, *18*, 65–87

Sarason, I. G. (1972) 'Experimental approaches to test anxiety: attention and the uses of information.' In C. D. Spielberger (ed), *Anxiety: current trends in theory and research*, vol 2, New York: Academic Press

—— (1978) 'The test anxiety scale: concept and research.' In C. D. Spielberger & I. G. Sarason (eds), *Stress and anxiety*, vol 5, New York: Hemisphere/Wiley

Sartorius, N. & Ban, T. A. (1986) *Assessment of depression.* Berlin: Springer-Verlag

Saunders, B. & Allsop, S. (1987) 'Relapse: a psychological perspective.' *British Journal of Addiction, 82*, 417–29

Saunders, W. M. & Kershaw, P. W. (1978) 'The prevalence of "problem drinking" and "alcoholism" in the West of Scotland.' *British Journal of Psychiatry, 133*, 493

——— & Kershaw, P. W. (1980) 'Screening test for alcoholism: findings from a community study.' *British Journal of Addiction, 75*, 37–41

——— & Richard, G. (1978) '"In vivo veritas"; an observational study of alcoholics' and normal drinkers' patterns of consumption.' *British Journal of Addiction, 73*, 375–80

Schooler, C. & Spohn, H. E. (1982) 'Social dysfunction and treatment failure in schizophrenia.' *Schizophrenia Bulletin, 8*, 85–98

Schuckitt, M. A. (1987) 'Biological vulnerability to alcoholism.' *Journal of Consulting and Clinical Psychology, 55*, 301–9

Schultz, H. T., Kelley, J., Overall, J. E. & Hollister, L. E. (1985) 'Factor structure of the drinking behaviour interview in a private inpatient treatment program.' *Journal of Studies on Alcohol, 46*, 132–6

Scott, R. R., Himadi, W. & Keane, T. M. (1983) 'A review of generalization in social skills training: suggestions for future research.' In M. Hersen, R. M. Eisler & P. Miller (eds), *Progress in Behavior Modification*, vol 15, New York: Academic Press

Segal, Z. V. & Shaw, B. F. (1986a) 'Cognition and depression: a reappraisal of Coyne and Gotlib's critique.' *Cognitive Therapy and Research, 10*, 671–93

——— & ——— (1986b) 'When cul-de-sacs are more mentality than reality: a rejoinder to Coyne and Gotlib.' *Cognitive Therapy and Research, 10*, 707–14

Selby, G. & Lance, J. W. (1960) 'Observations on 500 cases of migraine and allied vascular headache.' *Journal of Neurology, Neurosurgery and Psychiatry, 23*, 23

Seligman, M. E. P. (1975) *Helplessness: on depression, development, and death.* San Franciso: Freeman

———, Abramson, L. Y., Semmel, A. & von Bayer, C. (1979) 'Depressive attributional scale.' *Journal of Abnormal Psychology, 88*, 242–7

——— & Hager, J. L. (1972) *Biological boundaries of learning.* New York: Appleton-Century-Crofts

Seltzer, C. C. & Mayer, J. (1965) 'A simple criterion of obesity.' *Postgraduate Medicine, 38*, 101–7

Selzer, M. L. (1971) 'The Michigan alcoholism screening test: the quest for a new diagnostic instrument.' *American Journal of Psychiatry, 127*, 1653–8

———, Gomberg, E. S. & Nordhoff, J. A. (1979) 'Men and women's responses to the Michigan alcoholism screening test.' *Journal of Studies on Alcohol, 40*, 520–4

Senay, E. C. (1983) *Substance abuse disorders in clinical practice.* Boston: John Wright

Shaw, B. F. (1977) 'Comparison of cognitive therapy and behavior therapy in the treatment of depression.' *Journal of Consulting and Clinical Psychology, 45*, 543–51

Shealey, R. C., Lowe, J. D. & Ritzler, B. A. (1980) 'Sleep onset insomnia: personality characteristics and treatment outcome.' *Journal of Consulting and Clinical Psychology*, *48*, 659–61

Sheehan, D. V., Sheehan, K. E. & Minichiello, W. E. (1981) 'Age of onset of phobic disorders: a reevaluation.' *Comprehensive Psychiatry*, *22*, 544–53

Shelton, J., Hollister, L. E. & Gocka, E. F. (1969). 'The drinking behavior interview: an attempt to quantify alcohol impairment.' *Disorders of the Nervous System*, *30*, 464–7.

Shepherd, G. (1983a) Social skills training with adults: Preface. In S. Spence & G. Shepherd (eds), *Developments in social skills training*, London: Academic Press

——— (1983b) Introduction. Chapter 1. In S. H. Spence & G. Shepherd (eds), *Developments in social skills training*, London: Academic Press

Shiffman, S. (1982) 'Relapse following smoking cessation: a situational analysis.' *Journal of Consulting and Clinical Psychology*, *50*, 71–86

Silverstein, S. J., Nathan, P. E. & Taylor, H. A. (1974) 'Blood alcohol estimation and controlled drinking by chronic alcoholics.' *Behavior Therapy*, *5*, 1–15

Silverstone, T. & Turner, P. (1982) *Drug treatment in psychiatry*, 3rd edn, London: Routledge & Kegan Paul

Sisson, R. W. & Azrin, N. H. (1986) 'Family-member involvement to initiate and promote treatment of problem drinkers.' *Journal of Behavior Therapy and Experimental Psychiatry*, *17*, 15–21

Skinner, H. A. (1982) 'The drug abuse screening test.' *Addictive Behaviors*, *7*, 363–71

——— & Allen, B. A. (1982) 'Alcohol dependence syndrome: measurement and validation.' *Journal of Abnormal Psychology*, *91*, 199–209

———, Holt, S., Schuller, R., Roy, J. & Israel, Y. (1984) 'Identification of alcohol abuse using laboratory tests and a history of trauma.' *Annals of Internal Medicine*, *101*, 847–51

——— & Sheu, W. J. (1982) 'Reliability of alcohol use indices: the lifetime drinking history and the MAST.' *Journal of Studies on Alcohol*, *43*, 1157–70

Smith, M. E. & Fremouw, W. J. (1987) 'A realistic approach to treating obesity.' *Clinical Psychology Review*, *7*, 449–65

Sobell, M. B., Schaefer, H. H. & Mills, K. C. (1972) 'Differences in baseline drinking behaviour between alcoholics and social drinkers.' *Behaviour Research and Therapy*, *10*, 257–67

Solomon, R. L. (1980) 'An opponent-process theory of acquired motivation: the costs of pleasure and the benefits of pain.' *American Psychologist*, *35*, 691–712

Sorlie, P., Gordon, T. & Kanel, W. B. (1980) 'Body build and mortality: the Framington study.' *Journal of the American Medical Association*, *243*, 1828–31

Southwick, L., Steele, C., Marlatt, A. & Lindell, M. (1981) 'Alcohol-related expectancies: defined by phase of intoxication and drinking experience.' *Journal of Consulting and Clinical Psychology*, *49*, 713–21

Spanier, G. B. (1976) 'Measuring dyadic adjustment: new scales for assessing the quality of marriage and similar dyads.' *Journal of Marriage and the Family*, 15–29

Spence, S. H. (1983) 'The training of heterosexual social skills.' In S. H. Spence and G. Shepherd (eds), *Developments in social skills training*, London: Academic Press

——— (1985) 'Group versus individual treatment of primary and secondary female orgasmic dysfunction.' *Behaviour Research and Therapy*, *23*, 539–48

Spielberger, C. D., Gonzalez, H. P., Taylor, C. J., Algaze, B. & Anton, W. D. (1978) 'Examination stress and test anxiety.' In C. D. Spielberger & I. G. Sarason (eds), *Stress and anxiety*, vol 5, New York: Hemisphere/Wiley

———, Gorsuch, R. L., Lushene, R., Vagg, P. R. & Jacobs, G. A. (1983) *Manual for the state-trait anxiety inventory (Form Y). ('Self-evaluation questionnaire')*. Palo Alto, CA: Consulting Psychologists Press

Spitzer, R. L., Williams, J. B. W. & Gibbon, M. (1987) *Instruction manual for the structured clinical interview for DSM-III-R* (SCID; April 1987 Revision). New York: Biometrics Research Department, New York State Psychiatric Institute

Spivack, G. & Shure, M. B. (1976) *Social adjustment of young children: a cognitive approach to solving real life problems*. Jossey Bass: London

Stalonas, P. M., Johnson, W. G. & Christ, M. (1978) 'Behavior modification of obesity: the evaluation of exercise, contingency management and programme adherence.' *Journal of Consulting and Clinical Psychology*, *46*, 463–9

Steele, C. M., Southwick, L. & Pagano, R. (1986) 'Drinking your troubles away: the role of alcohol and activity.' *Journal of Abnormal Psychology*, *95*, 173–80

Stefanek, M. E. & Eisler, R. M. (1973) 'The current status of cognitive variables in assertion training.' In M. Hersen, R. Eisler & P. M. Miller (eds), *Progress in behavior modification*, vol 15, New York: Academic Press

Stern, J. S. (1984) 'Is obesity a disease of inactivity?' In A. J. Stunkard & E. Steller (eds), *Eating and its disorders*, New York: Raven Press

Stitzer, M. L., Bigelow, G. E. & McCaul, M. E. (1983) 'Behavioral approaches to drug abuse.' In M. Hersen, R. M. Eisler & P. M. Miller (eds), *Progress in behavior modification*, vol 14, New York: Academic Press, pp. 49–123

Stockwell, T., Hodgson, R., Edwards, G., Taylor, C. & Rankin, H. (1979) 'The development of a questionnaire to measure severity of alcohol dependence.' *British Journal of Addiction*, *74*, 79–87

———, Murphy, D. & Hodgson, R. (1983) 'The severity of alcohol dependence questionnaire: its use, reliability and validity.' *British Journal of Addiction*, *78*, 145–55

Stout, C., Morrow, J., Brandt, E. N. & Wolf, S. (1964) 'Unusually low incidence of death from myocardial infarction: study of an Italian American community in Pennsylvania.' *Journal of the American Medical Association*, *188*, 845–9

Strain, G. W., Strain, J. J., Zurnoff, B. & Knittle, J. (1984) 'Do fat cell morphometrics predict weight loss maintenance?' *International Journal of*

Obesity, *8*, 53–9
Stuart, R. B. & Davis, B. (1972) *Slim chance in a fat world: behavioral control of obesity*. Champaign, IL: Research Press
Stunkard, A. J. (1983) 'Biological and psychological factors in obesity.' In K. Goodstein (ed), *Eating and weight disorders*, New York: Springer
——— & Koch, C. (1964) 'The interpretation of gastric mobility: apparent bias in the reports of hunger by obese persons.' *Archives of General Psychiatry*, *11*, 74–82
——— & Mazer, A. (1978) 'Smorgasbord and obesity.' *Psychosomatic Medicine*, *40*, 173–5
———, Sorensen, T. I., Hanis, C., Teasdale, T. W., Chakrabarty, R., Schull, W. J. & Schulsinger, F. (1986) 'An adoption study of human obesity.' *New England Journal of Medicine*, *314*, 193–8
Sturgis, E. T. & Arena, J. G. (1984) 'Psychophysiological assessment.' In M. Hersen, R. M. Eisler & P. M. Miller (eds), *Progress in behavior modification*, vol 17, New York: Academic Press
Suinn, R. M. (1969) 'The STABS, a measure of test anxiety for behavior therapy: normative data.' *Behaviour Research and Therapy*, *7*, 335–9
Supnick, J. A. & Coletti, G. (1984) 'Relapse coping and problem solving training following treatment for smoking.' *Addictive Behaviors*, *9*, 401–4
Sussman, S., Rychtarik, R. G., Mueser, K., Glynn, S. & Prue, D. M. (1986) 'Ecological relevance of memory tests and the prediction of relapse in alcoholics.' *Journal of Studies on Alcohol*, *47*, 305–10
Sutherland, G., Edwards, G., Taylor, C., Phillips, G., Gossop, M. & Brady, R. (1986) 'The measurement of opiate dependence.' *British Journal of Addiction*, *81*, 485–94
Swenson, W. M. & Morse, R. M. (1975) 'The use of a self-administered alcoholism screening test (SAAST) in a medical center.' *Mayo Clinic Proceedings*, *50*, 204–8
Tan, D. L., Kales, J. D., Kales, A., Soldatos, C. R. & Bixler, E. O. (1987) 'Biopsychobehavioral correlates of insomnia, IV: diagnosis based on the DSM-III.' *American Journal of Psychiatry*, *141*, 357–62
Taylor, C. B. & Agras, S. (1981) 'Assessment of phobia.' In D. H. Barlow (ed), *Behavioral assessment of adult disorders*, New York: Guilford Press, pp. 181–208
Taylor, J. A. (1953) 'A personality scale of manifest anxiety.' *Journal of Abnormal and Social Psychology*, *48*, 285–90
Teasdale, J. D. (1983) 'Negative thinking in depression: cause, effect, or reciprocal relationship?' *Advances in Behaviour Research and Therapy*, *5*, 3–25
Thompson, J. K. (1982) 'Diagnosis of head pain: an ideographic approach to assessment of head and facial pain.' *Headache*, *22*, 211
——— & Figueroa, J. (1983) 'Critical issues in the assessment of headache.' In M. Hersen, R. M. Eisler & P. M. Miller (eds), *Progress in behavior modification*, vol 15, New York: Academic Press
Thomson, I. G. & Rathod, N. H. (1968) 'Aversion therapy for heroin dependence.' *The Lancet*, 382–4
Thyer, B. A., Papsdorf, J. D., Davis, R. & Vallecorsa, S. (1984) 'Autonomic correlates of the subjective anxiety scale.' *Journal of Behavior*

Therapy and Experimental Psychiatry, *15*, 3–7
Tiffany, S. T., Martin, E. M. & Baker, T. B. (1986) 'Treatments for cigarette smoking: an evaluation of the contributions of aversive and counseling procedures.' *Behaviour Research and Therapy*, *24*, 437–52
Tinklenberg, J. R. (1973) 'Alcohol and violence.' In P. G. Bourne and R. Fox (eds), *Alcoholism: progress in research and treatment*, New York: Academic Press, pp. 195–210
Tokarz, T. & Lawrence, P. (1974) 'An analysis of temporal and stimulus factors in the treatment of insomnia.' Paper presented at the meeting of the Association for the Advancement of Behavior Therapy, Chicago
Tomlin, P., Thyer, B. A., Curtis, G. C., Nesse, R., Cameron, O. & Wright, P. (1984) 'Standardization of the fear survey schedule based upon patients with DSM-III anxiety disorders.' *Journal of Behavior Therapy and Experimental Psychiatry*, *15*, 123–6
Torgerson, S. (1983) 'Genetic factors in anxiety disorders.' *Archives of General Psychiatry*, *40*, 1085–92
Trimmer, E. (1978) 'Reducing the side effects of the pill.' *British Journal of Sexual Medicine*, *5*, 62–70
Trower, P. (1984) *Radical approaches to social skills training*. London: Croom Helm
———, Bryant, B. & Argyle, M. (1978) *Social skills and mental health*. London: Methuen
———, Yardley, K., Bryant, B. & Shaw, P. (1978) 'The treatment of social failure: a comparison of anxiety reduction and skills acquisition procedures on two social problems.' *Behavior Modification*, *2*, 41–60
Truax, C. & Carkuff, R. (1967) *Toward effective counselling and psychotherapy*. Chicago: Aldine
Tryon, G. S. (1980) 'The measurement and treatment of test anxiety.' *Review of Educational Research*, *50*, 343–72
Turner, R. M. & Ascher, L. M. (1979) 'Controlled comparison of progressive relaxation, stimulus control, and paradoxical intention therapies for insomnia.' *Journal of Consulting and Clinical Psychology*, *47*, 500–8
Turner, S. M. (ed) (1984) *Behavioral theories and treatment of anxiety*. New York: Plenum
Tyler, L. (1969) *The work of the counselor*, 3rd edn, Englewood Cliffs, NJ: Prentice-Hall
Van Dam-Baggen, R. & Kraaimaat, F. (1986) 'A group social skills training programme with psychiatric patients: outcome, drop-out rate and prediction.' *Behaviour Research and Therapy*, *24*, 161–9
Van Hasselt, V. B., Hersen, M. & Milliones, J. (1978) 'Social skills training for alcoholics and drug addicts: a review.' *Addictive Behaviors*, *3*, 221–33
Van Itallie, T. B. (1979) 'Obesity: adverse effects on health and longevity.' *American Journal of Clinical Nutrition*, *32*, 2723–33
Vandereycken, W. (1983) 'Agoraphobia and marital relationship: theory, treatment, and research.' *Clinical Psychology Review*, *31*, 317–38
Veleber, D. M. & Templer, D. I. (1984) 'Effects of caffeine on anxiety and depression.' *Journal of Abnormal Psychology*, *93*, 120–22
Voegtlin, W. L. (1940) 'The treatment of alcoholism by establishing a

conditioned reflex.' *American Journal of the Medical Sciences, 199*, 802–10

Vogt, T., Selvin, S., Widdowson, G. & Hulley, S. B. (1977) 'Expired air carbon monoxide and serum thiocyanate as objective measures of cigarette exposure.' *American Journal of Public Health, 67*, 545–9

Wadden, T. A. & Stunkard, A. J. (1986) 'Controlled trial of very low calorie diet, behaviour therapy and their combination in the treatment of obesity.' *Journal of Consulting and Clinical Psychology, 54*, 482–8

Walk, R. D. (1956) 'Self ratings of fear in a fear-invoking situation.' *Journal of Abnormal and Social Psychology, 52*, 171–8

Wallace, C. J., Nelson, C. H., Liberman, R. P., Aitchison, R. A., Lukoff, D., Elder, J. P. & Ferris, C. (1980) 'A review and critique of social skills training with schizophrenic patients.' *Schizophrenia Bulletin, 6*, 42–62

Wanberg, K. W., Horn, J. L. & Foster, F. M. (1977) 'A differential assessment model for alcoholism: the scales of the alcohol use inventory.' *Journal of Studies on Alcohol, 38*, 512–43

Watson, D. & Friend, R. (1969) 'Measurement of social-evaluative anxiety.' *Journal of Consulting and Clinical Psychology, 33*, 448–57

Watson, J. M. (1980) 'Solvent abuse by children and young adults: a review.' *British Journal of Addiction, 75*, 27–36

Watts, F. N. & Sherrock, R. (1984) 'Questionnaire dimensions of spider phobia.' *Behaviour Research and Therapy, 22*, 575–80

Webster, A. S. (1953) 'The development of phobias in married women.' *Psychological Monographs, 67*, 1–18

Weiss, A. R. (1977) 'A behavioral approach to the treatment of adolescent obesity.' *Behavior Therapy, 8*, 720–6

Weiss, E. (ed) (1964) *Agoraphobia in the light of ego psychology*. New York: Grune & Stratton

Weiss, J. M., Glazer, H. I., Pohorecky, L., Brick, J. & Miller, N. E. (1975) 'Effects of chronic exposure to stressors on avoidance-escape behavior and on brain norepinephrine.' *Psychosomatic Medicine, 37*, 522–33

———, Stone, E. A. & Harrell, N. (1970) 'Coping behavior and brain norepinephrine level in rats.' *Journal of Comparative and Physiological Psychology, 72*, 153–60

Weissman, A. N. & Beck, A. T. (1978) 'Development and validation of the dysfunctional attitudes scale.' Paper presented at the American Educational Research Association Annual Convention, Toronto, Canada

Whitehead, E. D., Klyde, B. J., Zussman, S., Wayne, N., Shinbach, K. & Davis, D. (1983) 'Male sexual dysfunction and diabetes mellitus.' *New York State Journal of Medicine, 83*, 1174–9

Whitfield, J. B., Hensley, W. J., Bryden, D. & Gallagher, H. (1978) 'Some laboratory correlates of drinking habits.' *Annals of Clinical Biochemistry, 15*, 297–303

Wilkins, R. (1974) *The hidden alcoholic in general practice*. London: Elek Science

Wilkinson, D. A. & Sanchez-Craig, M. A. (1981) 'Relevance of brain dysfunction to treatment objectives: should alcohol-related cognitive deficits change the way we think about treatment?' *Addictive Behaviors*, *6*, 253–60

Wilkinson, I. M. & Blackburn, I. M. (1981) 'Cognitive style in depressed and recovered depressed patients.' *British Journal of Clinical Psychology*, *20*, 283–92

Williams, J. M. G. (1984) *The psychological treatment of depression: a guide to the theory and practice of cognitive-behavior therapy*, London: Croom Helm

Williams, S. L. & Rappoport, A. (1983) 'Cognitive treatment in the natural environment for agoraphobics.' *Behavior Therapy*, *14*, 299–313

——— & Watson, N. (1985) 'Perceived danger and perceived self-efficacy as cognitive determinants of acrophobic behavior.' *Behavior Therapy*, *16*, 136–46

Williamson, D. A. (1981) 'Behavioural treatment of migraine and muscle-contraction headaches: outcome and theoretical explanations.' In M. Hersen, R. M. Eisler & P. M. Miller (eds), *Progress in behavior modification*, vol 11, New York: Academic Press

Wilson, G. T. (1987) 'Cognitive studies in alcoholism.' *Journal of Consulting and Clinical Psychology*, *55*, 325–31

Wilson, P. H. & Forbes, M. (1987) 'The insomnia cognitions scale.' Unpublished manuscript, University of Sydney

———, Goldin, J. C. & Charbonneau-Powis, M. (1983) 'Comparative efficacy of behavioral and cognitive treatments of depression.' *Cognitive Therapy and Research*, *7*, 111–24

Wincze, J. P. (1982) 'Assessment of sexual disorders.' *Behavioral Assessment*, *4*, 257–71

Wolfe, J., Keane, T. M., Lyons, J. A. & Geraldi, R. J. (1987) 'Current trends and issues in the assessment of combat-related post-traumatic stress disorder.' *The Behavior Therapist*, *10*, 27–32

Wolpe, J. (1958) *Psychotherapy by reciprocal inhibition*. Stanford: Stanford University Press

——— (1969) *The practice of behavior therapy*, 1st edn, New York: Pergamon Press

——— & Lang, P. J. (1964) 'A fear survey schedule for use in behavior therapy.' *Behavior Research and Therapy*, *2*, 27–30

——— & ——— (1969) *Fear Survey Schedule*. San Diego, CA: Educational and Industrial Testing Service

——— & Lazarus, A. A. (1966) *Behavior Therapy Techniques*. New York: Pergamon Press

Wooley, S. C., Wooley, O. W. & Dyrenforth, E. R. (1979) 'Theoretical, practical and social issues in behavioral treatment of obesity.' *Journal of Applied Behavior Analysis*, *12*, 3–26

Wynne, L. C. & Solomon, R. L. (1955) 'Traumatic avoidance in learning: acquisition and extinction in dogs deprived of normal peripheral autonomic function.' *Genetic Psychology Monographs*, *52*, 241–84

Yates, A. J. & Thain, J. (1985) 'Self-efficacy as a predictor of relapse following voluntary cessation of smoking.' *Addictive Behaviors*, *10*, 291–8

Young, M. A., Scheftner, W. A., Klerman, G. L., Andreasen, N. C. & Hirschfield, R. M. (1986) 'The endogenous subtype of depression: a study of its internal construct validity.' *British Journal of Psychiatry*, *148*, 257–67

Young, M. (1982) 'The role of expectancy in the behavioural treatment of insomnia.' Master of Psychology thesis, University of New South Wales

Young, R. M. & Knight, R. G. (1986) 'The drinking expectancy questionnaire: a measure of alcohol related beliefs.' Unpublished manuscript, University of Queensland

Youngren, M. A. & Lewinsohn, P. M. (1980) 'The functional relation between depression and problematic interpersonal behavior.' *Journal of Abnormal Psychology*, *89*, 333–41

Zafiropoulou, M. & McPherson, F. M. (1986) ' "Preparedness" and the severity and outcome of clinical phobias.' *Behaviour Research and Therapy*, *24*, 221–2

Ziegler, D. K., Hassanein, R. S. & Couch, J. R. (1977) 'Characteristics of life headache histories in a non-clinic population.' *Neurology*, *27*, 265–9

Zigler, E. & Phillips, L. (1961) 'Social competence and outcome in mental disorder.' *Journal of Abnormal Psychology*, *63*, 264–71

Zimmerman, M. & Coryell, W. (1987) 'The inventory to diagnose depression (IDD): a self-report scale to diagnose major depressive disorder.' *Journal of Consulting and Clinical Psychology*, *55*, 55–9

———, Coryell, W., Pfohl, B. & Stangl, D. A. (1986) 'The validity of four definitions of endogenous depression II: clinical, demographic, familial, and psychosocial correlates.' *Archives of General Psychiatry*, *43*, 234–44

Zung, W. W. K. (1965) 'A self-rating depression scale.' *Archives of General Psychiatry*, *12*, 63–70

——— & Cavenar, J. O. (1980) 'Assessment scales and techniques.' In I. L. Kutash, L. B. Schlesinger *et al.* (eds), *Handbook on stress and anxiety*, San Francisco, CA: Jossey-Bass, pp. 348–63

Zwart, C. A. & Lisman, S. A. (1979) 'Analysis of stimulus control treatment of sleep-onset insomnia.' *Journal of Consulting and Clinical Psychology*, *47*, 113–18

Author Index

Author Index

Subject Index

For Product Safety Concerns and Information please contact our EU representative GPSR@taylorandfrancis.com
Taylor & Francis Verlag GmbH, Kaufingerstraße 24, 80331 München, Germany

www.ingramcontent.com/pod-product-compliance
Ingram Content Group UK Ltd.
Pitfield, Milton Keynes, MK11 3LW, UK
UKHW022156190926
475702UK00003B/49
* 9 7 8 1 1 3 8 3 2 4 7 2 5 *